Innovations in Pilates
Matwork
for Health and Wellbeing

Anthony Lett / Kenyi Diaz

First published December 2015
Text © Innovations in Pilates, 2015
Published by Innovations in Pilates
with the assistance of Rebus Press

Innovations in Pilates
Level One, 175 Brunswick Street
Fitzroy VIC 3065
Australia
info@innovationsinpilates.com.au
www.innovationsinpilates.com.au

Rebus Press
PO Box 622
Hurstbridge VIC 3099
Email: julie@rebuspress.com.au
Web: www.rebuspress.com.au

Photography by Gabriela Medina, www.gabrielamedina.com
Anatomy diagrams used with permission of Muscle and Motion
Cover design by Kenyi Diaz
Layout by Kenyi Diaz
Modelling by Kenyi Diaz, Hilse Leon and Anthony Lett

ISBN: 978-0-9945147-0-7 (CD Rom)

All rights reserved. No part of this book may be reproduced or transmitted in any form or by any means, electronic or mechanical, including photocopying, recording or by any information storage and retrieval system, without written permission from the publisher, except for the inclusion of brief quotations in a review.

The author and publisher have taken care in the preparation of this CD but make no expressed or implied warranty of any kind and assume no responsibility for errors or omissions. No liability is assumed for incidental or consequential damages in connection with or arising out of the use of the information or programs contained herein.

Contents

Foreword vii

Part A – Classical Exercises

Introduction – Part A 2
Part A Planes of Movement 4
Part A Matwork – Classical Exercises 6
1 The Hundred 8
2 The Roll Up 9
3 The Roll Over 10
4 Rolling Back 11
5 One Leg Circle 12
6 One Leg Stretch 13
7 Double Leg Stretch 14
8 Spine Stretch 15
9 Rocker with Open legs 16
10 The Cork Screw 17
11 The Saw 18
12 Swan Dive 19
13 One Leg Kick 20
14 Double Leg Kick 21
15 Neck Pull 22
16 Scissors 23
17 The Bicycle 24
18 Shoulder Bridge 25
19 Spine Twist 26
20 Jack Knife 27
21 Side Kick 28
22 The Teaser 29
23 Hip Twist with Stretched Arms 30
24 Swimming 31
25 Leg Pull Front 32
26 Leg Pull 33
27 Side Kick Kneeling 34
28 Side Bend 35
29 The Seal 36
30 Rocking 37
31 Control Balance 38
32 Push Up 39

Part B – Innovations Stretches

Introduction – Part B 41
Compression – the Shoulder Joint 51
Compression – the Hip Joint 52
Compression – the Lumbar Spine 53

The Calves/Lower Leg/Foot

Chapter 1 – Muscle Chart 55
1 Seated Toe Extension 57

    2 Standing Calf. 58
    3 Lying Calf with Strap. 59
    4 One Leg Dog Pose 60
    4 One Leg Dog Pose 61
    5 Toe Flexion 62
    6 Seated Tibialis Anterior 63
    7 Floor Tibialis Anterior 64
    8 Seated Inversion. 65
    9 Inversion with Strap 66
    10 Seated Eversion 67
    11 Eversion with Strap 68

The Hamstrings
    Chapter 2 – Muscle Chart. 70
    12 Foam Roller Hamstring 71
    13 Hamstring Glute Exploration 72
    14 Hamstring Glute Partner 73
    15 Lying Medial and Lateral 74
    16 Lying Straight Leg Hamstring 75
    17 The Mex Stretch 76
    18 Seated Bent-Leg Hamstring 77
    19 Seated Calf, Hamstring Partner 78

The Hip Flexors and Quadriceps
    Chapter 3 – Muscle Chart. 80
    20 Foam Roller Hamstrings Glute 81
    21 Kneeling Quadriceps Box 82
    22 Kneeling Hip Flexors 83
    23 Lying Quadricep 84
    23 Lying Quadricep Variation 85
    24 Standing Quadricep 86
    25 Floor Godzilla. 87
    26 Lunge Pose 88
    26 Lunge Pose Variation. 89

The Gluteal Region
    Chapter 4 – Muscle Chart. 91
    27 Seated Hip 92
    28 Criss Cross 93
    29 Box Pigeon 94
    30 Box Twist 95
    31 Pigeon. 96

The Adductors
    Chapter 5 – Muscle Chart. 98
    32 The Frog. 99
    33 Kneeling Short Long 100
    34 Lying Adductors 101
    35 Seated Partner Adductors. 102
    36 Seated Bent Leg Split 103

The Trunk

    Chapter 6 – Muscle Chart 105
    37 The Accelerator 106
    38 The Dangler. 107
    39 The Cat 108
    40 Hamstring Spine Combo. 109
    41 BOSU Back Bend 110
    42 The Cobra. 111
    43 Box Wheel 112
    44 Floor Wheel 113
    45 Seated Rotation 114
    46 Lying Rotation 115
    47 Car Crash 116
    48 Pull and Push 117
    49 Foam Roller Mermaid 118
    50 Floor Side Bend. 119
    51 Seated Side Bend. 120
    52 Seated Side Bend Variation 121

The Chest, Arms and Shoulders

    Chapter 7 – Muscle Chart 123
    Chapter 7 – Muscle Chart 124
    53 Box Lats. 126
    54 Foam Roller Pectoralis Stretch 127
    55 Lying Pectoralis Major. 128
    56 Lying Bicep 129
    57 Standing Pectoralis Minor 130
    58 Tricep/Lats 131
    59 Partner Internal Rotators 132
    60 Partner External Rotators 133
    61 Stick Internal Rotators 134
    62 Forearm Extensors. 135
    63 Forearm Flexors 136
    64 Pronators. 137

The Neck

    Chapter 8 – Muscle Chart 139
    66 Neck Flexion 140
    67 Neck Flexion and Rotation. 141
    68 Neck Lateral Flexion 142
    69 Neck Rotation 143
    70 Neck Extension and Rotation 144
    71 Jaw Extension 145

The Split

    72 The Split. 147
    Some recommendations on how to use this book 148
    Concluding Comments 149
    Bibliography 150

Foreword

By Rael Isacowitz
Founder BASI Pilates

The Pilates industry needs innovators and forward-thinkers like Mr Anthony Lett. Since I first met Anthony in 2011 he has never ceased to display creativity, intelligence and a never-ending abundance of new ideas. *Innovations in Pilates: Matwork for Health and Wellbeing* is another of Anthony's well thought out and beautifully presented books. It brings new dimensions of understanding to the Pilates Matwork and will no doubt contribute to the professional's and enthusiast's knowledge and enjoyment of the Matwork.

Mr Lett's specific focus on flexibility is enlightening, and his breaking down the classic Pilates repertoire and the flexibility requirements of each exercise will prove extremely helpful to all who practice Pilates, be it on the mat or apparatus. Most importantly, *Innovations in Pilates: Matwork for Health and Wellbeing* will provide a road map for the safe practice of Pilates. Although Pilates is commonly thought of as a very safe system of exercise, and in the hands of well-educated teachers and practitioners it is, Pilates can also be damaging if certain basic physical requirements, one of them being adequate flexibility, are not present and the exercises are not well understood.

Anthony has used the original/classic Pilates exercises as performed and taught by Mr Joseph Pilates as the foundation and springboard for his work. This is an approach that was used in *Pilates Anatomy (Human Kinetics)* a widely distributed book authored by my colleague Karen Clippinger and I. It proved to be very valuable for a broad spectrum of the population that practices Pilates. I am certain Anthony will share the same success. He deconstructs the exercises into smaller movements making them easier to digest and perform. Many of the Pilates exercises are very complex and this system of deconstruction will no doubt provide valuable stepping-stones in the learning process. He then offers stretches to help achieve optimum performance of each exercise. These stretches are based on the most contemporary exercise science and research to be both safe and effective. The stretches include both individual and partner stretches. The book is exquisitely illustrated and each illustration conveys layer upon layer of information.

I have been practicing Pilates since the late 1970s and had the pleasure and honor of studying with several of Joseph Pilates first generation teachers, most notably Kathy Stanford-Grant. I am the founder and director of BASI Pilates, an international Pilates education company established in 1989, and I have been teaching and presenting around the globe for the past 30 years. Anthony and I share a strong belief and drive to provide the highest level of postgraduate education for Pilates professionals from all backgrounds. BASI Pilates will now offer a Certificate Course, Pilates Anatomy, which has been compiled by Mr Lett. Anthony serves as the Director of Advanced education for BASI Pilates.

I am confident that *Innovations in Pilates: Matwork for Health and Wellbeing* will enhance anyone's practice of Pilates, but more importantly it will offer a path to wellbeing with unhindered and unrestricted movement in daily life – our ultimate goal.

Part A
Classical Exercises

Introduction – Part A

"Constantly keep in mind that you are not interested in developing merely bulging muscles, but rather flexible ones."

Joseph Pilates

WHAT? ANOTHER PILATES BOOK?

Before Kenyi and I undertook the considerable effort of producing this book, we needed to clarify why it was necessary. After all, bookshelves are flooded with Pilates books and DVDs. As teachers of Pilates, and teachers of Pilates teachers, we felt the area of flexibility development needed attention and warranted writing about. In the first book of this series, *Innovations in Pilates: Therapeutic Muscle Stretching on the Pilates Reformer,* I made a similar argument. I wrote about the history of Pilates and my experience, both personally and with others in the worldwide Pilates community, that although Joseph Pilates was a visionary and created his method to increase flexibility, advances in the areas of sport and medical science could be used to augment his work in this domain. Indeed, the stretching aspect of Joseph Pilates' original work has undergone little development in the years since the original set of exercises was developed. It seemed to me that the subject areas of core strength, neuromuscular development, cardiovascular and general strength in Pilates have been, and continue to be, the subject of much investigation and development in the exercise and medical science communities; whereas the subject of stretching seems to have slipped under the radar to some extent. We want to address this omission. Like Joseph Pilates, we believe that flexibility is an important physical attribute and we want ensure that the work experienced in any Pilates studio fulfils Joe's goal by keeping abreast of modern developments.

PRE-PILATES

"Civilization impairs physical fitness." J Pilates

In recent years, the original Pilates repertoire has been broken down (deconstructed if you will) into more simple movements known as "Pre-Pilates". Physiotherapists in Australia have developed "Clinical Pilates", a vastly pared-down version of the original for the treatment of injury. This deconstruction has occurred for two principal reasons. One, advances in knowledge have seen the Pilates community decide certain principles are key, and need further attention before a fuller, more complex movement like one of the original exercises can be attempted. Two, Joe's statement about civilisation rings true today even more strongly than ever before. Many in today's sedentary Western population are simply not up to the task of completing Joe's original work, especially not safely. Interestingly though, what is known as Pre-Pilates doesn't offer much in the way of stretching. And yet to perform the original work, a better than average degree of flexibility is required. So as well as developing this work to pay homage to one of Joe Pilates' original principles, we feel that some preliminary stretching is necessary in order for his original work to be performed safely and successfully.

RECOMMENDATIONS FOR USING THIS BOOK

In *Innovations in Pilates* I wrote about the use of the Pilates reformer as an exquisite piece of machinery for flexibility development. In this book we take a different approach. In Part A we look at the major flexibility requirements of the original 32 mat-based exercises (there are actually 34, but we have omitted two for safety reasons), first by demonstrating them, and then by breaking down the movements at each of the major joints and muscles involved in the exercise. We then direct you to particular stretches so you will be better able to perform the original work. More importantly, you will be more able to engage in the activities of daily life with the "spontaneous zest and pleasure" (J Pilates, *Your Health*) that Pilates himself had in mind for you. We call these preparatory stretches "facilitating stretches", as they make the original work more accessible and your performance of it safer, more effective and more graceful. (This is not to be confused with the practice of neuromuscular stretching called facilitated stretching). In part B we show you how to stretch all of the major muscle groups of your body, from the feet up. If you don't practise Pilates exercise, this section will keep you (as Joe Pilates used to say) "as supple as a cat". When you have mastered many of these exercises, you might be tempted to revisit Part A and try your hand (and body) at some of the Pilates classics. It is likely, therefore, that you will regularly flick, or click, between Parts A and B.

If an exercise does not have any particular flexibility requirements, for example the "Hundred", we will suggest counterposes. A counterpose is a stretch, an "antidote" movement, or group of stretches done to ensure that you do not become overly stiff with repeated performances of a particular exercise or movement pattern. Repeated performance of any exercise or movement – be it the Hundred, a tennis stroke or cycling – can bring about stiffness. Joe Pilates referred to such counterposes as "companion" exercises. In *Your Health* (p. 44) he writes, "The law of natural exercises recognizes companion or reciprocal movements in the normal development of the body."

If you are a Pilates devotee, read through Part A and explore on the mat or with your teacher those areas in which you experience difficulty performing the work. Chances are the stretches recommended will hit the spot for you. Once you identify your flexibility needs and follow our recommendations, your performance of the Pilates work will benefit tremendously. You will experience a certain poise and ease of movement during your Pilates classes that will persist past the session into your daily activities. This is important, of course, because we spend at most several hours of our week on the exercise mat. This transference into the "activities of daily life" (ADLs) is one of the chief goals of all of our exercise routines. Indeed, JP too was aware of the importance of transference, saying, "physical fitness is a uniformly developed body capable of performing our daily tasks naturally and easily, with spontaneous zest and pleasure." Today in particular, "functional fitness" has become the buzzword and focus of training. In rehabilitation domains like physiotherapy, all exercises are directed toward a return to ADLs. One caution though, don't forget the simple joy of movement in itself, irrespective of any later rewards that may accrue.

Of course, it must be acknowledged that not everyone is stiff, and if you have done years of yoga or dance for example, and come to Pilates with considerable flexibility, it may be that control and precision, two of the other important Pilates principles, are what's needed in your practice. If this is the case, we're sure you will find at least some of the stretches effective. One, because they are precise and will target some of the smaller muscles that are often left untouched in larger full-body, multi-joint movements like those practised in yoga or dance. And two, because the deep stretching we advocate will awaken you to the patterns of tension and flexibility and the sensations held within your body. This experience will develop a certain "body-mindfulness" that can have a hugely beneficial impact on your way of being and experiencing the world.

Finally, we know that repeated patterns of movement performed within a certain range, as in dance for example, will likely only maintain your flexibility and not increase it. In other cases, as with running, it will reduce your flexibility. So work with the stretches and find your tight spots, even if they exist within a mostly lithe body. As I am fond of quoting in my workshops, "We are the authors of ourselves. Through our actions, and our failure to act, we ultimately design ourselves". (Sartre). You will undoubtedly find this to be true for you, too. Whatever your personal history, use Part B to maintain or increase your current range of movement, your posture and grace, your mental focus, your awareness and your elegance. Enjoy the practice!

CLASSICAL OR CONTEMPORARY?

With the development of any method or technique, there will be differing interpretations on how the original ought to be performed, and a movement by some towards a more contemporary approach. If you favour a classical approach the flexibility requirements for your performance may differ from those of a contemporary practitioner. We ask you to respect these differences, and recognise that we cannot provide for every interpretation of every exercise in our book.

WHAT THIS BOOK IS NOT

While we expect that reading this book will improve your understanding of the Pilates mat work, it won't teach you how to perform the mat exercises. Our goal is to look at the flexibility requirements necessary to perform these exercises. To this end, we have analysed them in a fairly dry manner, devoid of colorful cues and giving only those details necessary to facilitate a better and safer performance of the work, regardless of the lineage of your teacher or training school.

Part A Planes of Movement

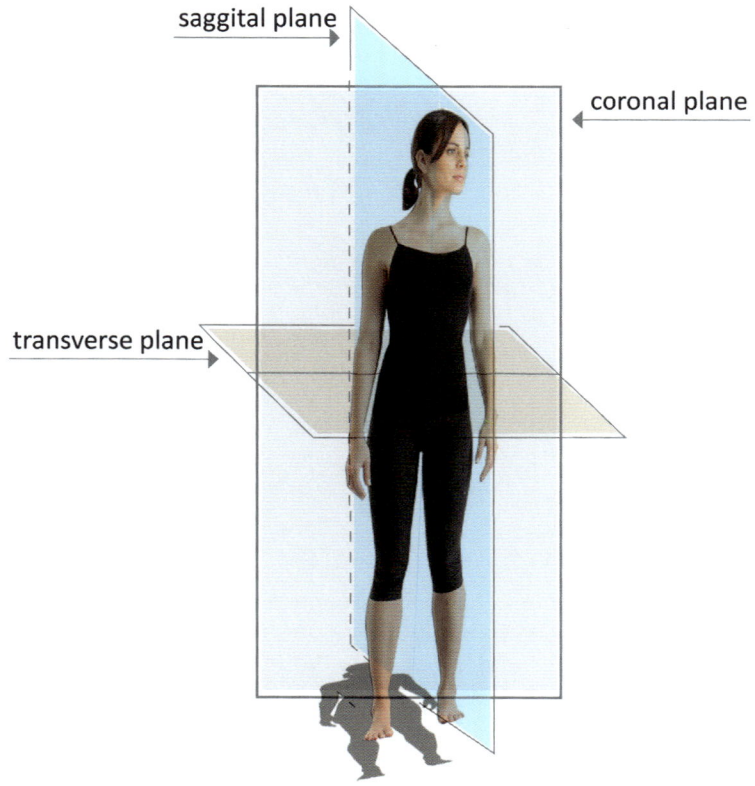

While this text is not intended to teach anatomy, we do use some basic anatomical descriptions of movement. If you are new to the terminology, refer to the illustrations when reading the breakdown of limb and joint movements in Part A. For example, when you read **"the shoulder is in flexion"** you can refer back to the illustrations to clarify what is meant.

Movements such as **"ulnar deviation"** and **"pronation"** have been left out because that level of detail is not necessary in this text.

Saggital plane: flexion and extension

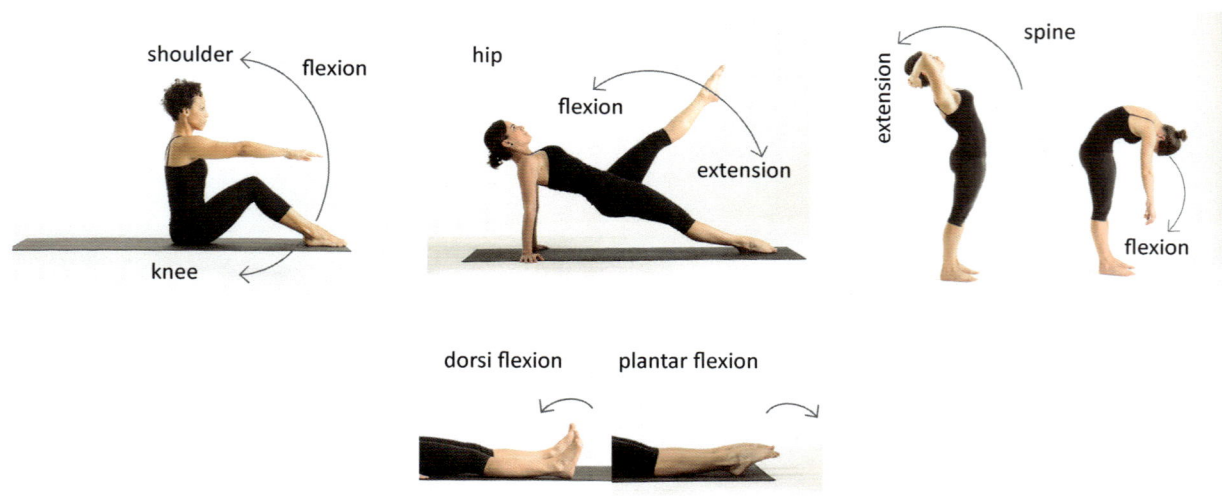

Coronal plane: adduction, abduction and lateral flexion

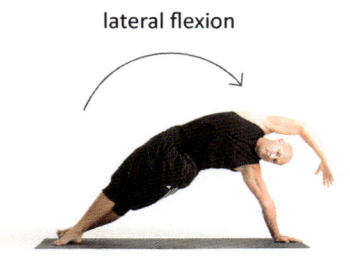
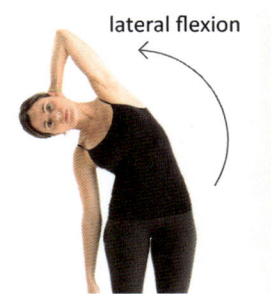
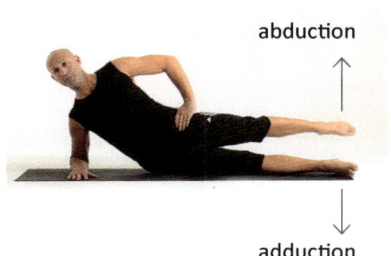

Transverse plane: rotation

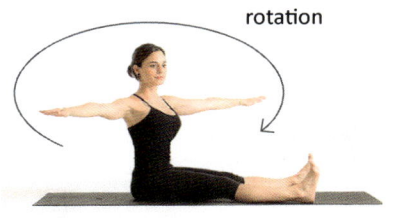
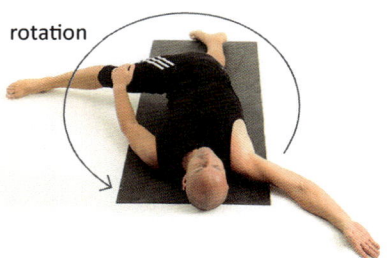

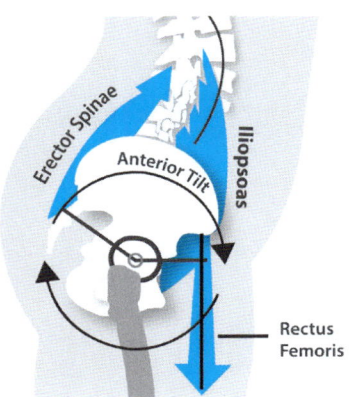
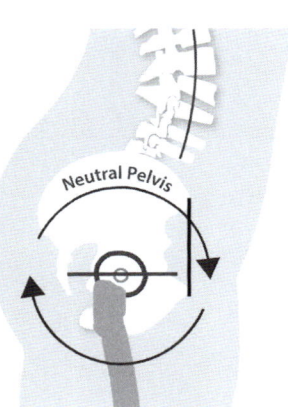
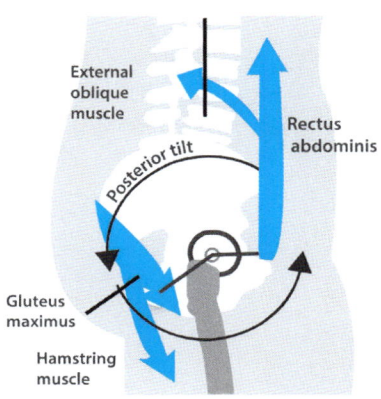

Anterior tilt   **Neutral pelvis**   **Posterior tilt**

Part A Matwork – Classical Exercises

"Contrology was conceived to limber and stretch muscles so that you will be as supple as a cat."
Joseph Pilates

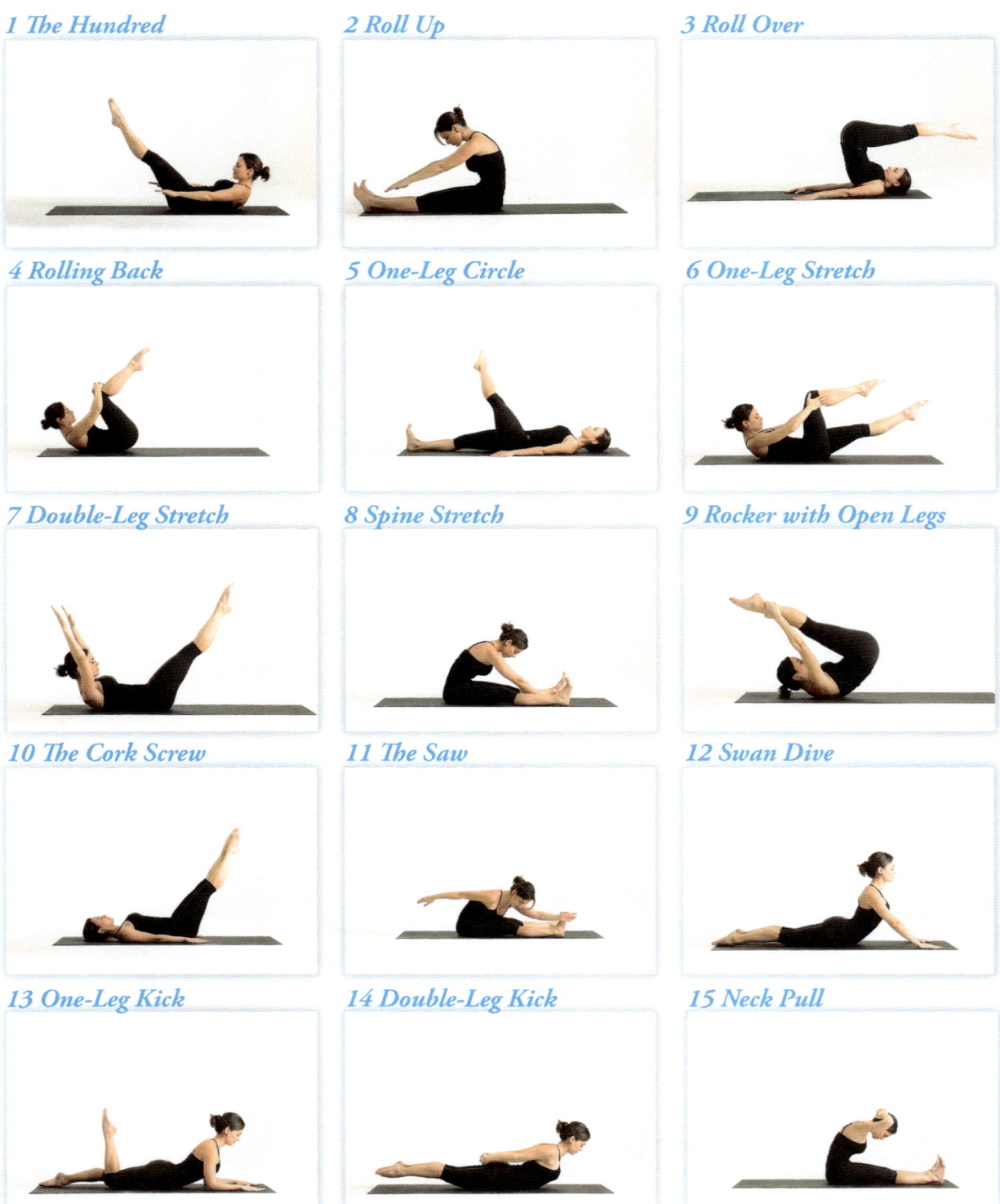

1 The Hundred
2 Roll Up
3 Roll Over
4 Rolling Back
5 One-Leg Circle
6 One-Leg Stretch
7 Double-Leg Stretch
8 Spine Stretch
9 Rocker with Open Legs
10 The Cork Screw
11 The Saw
12 Swan Dive
13 One-Leg Kick
14 Double-Leg Kick
15 Neck Pull

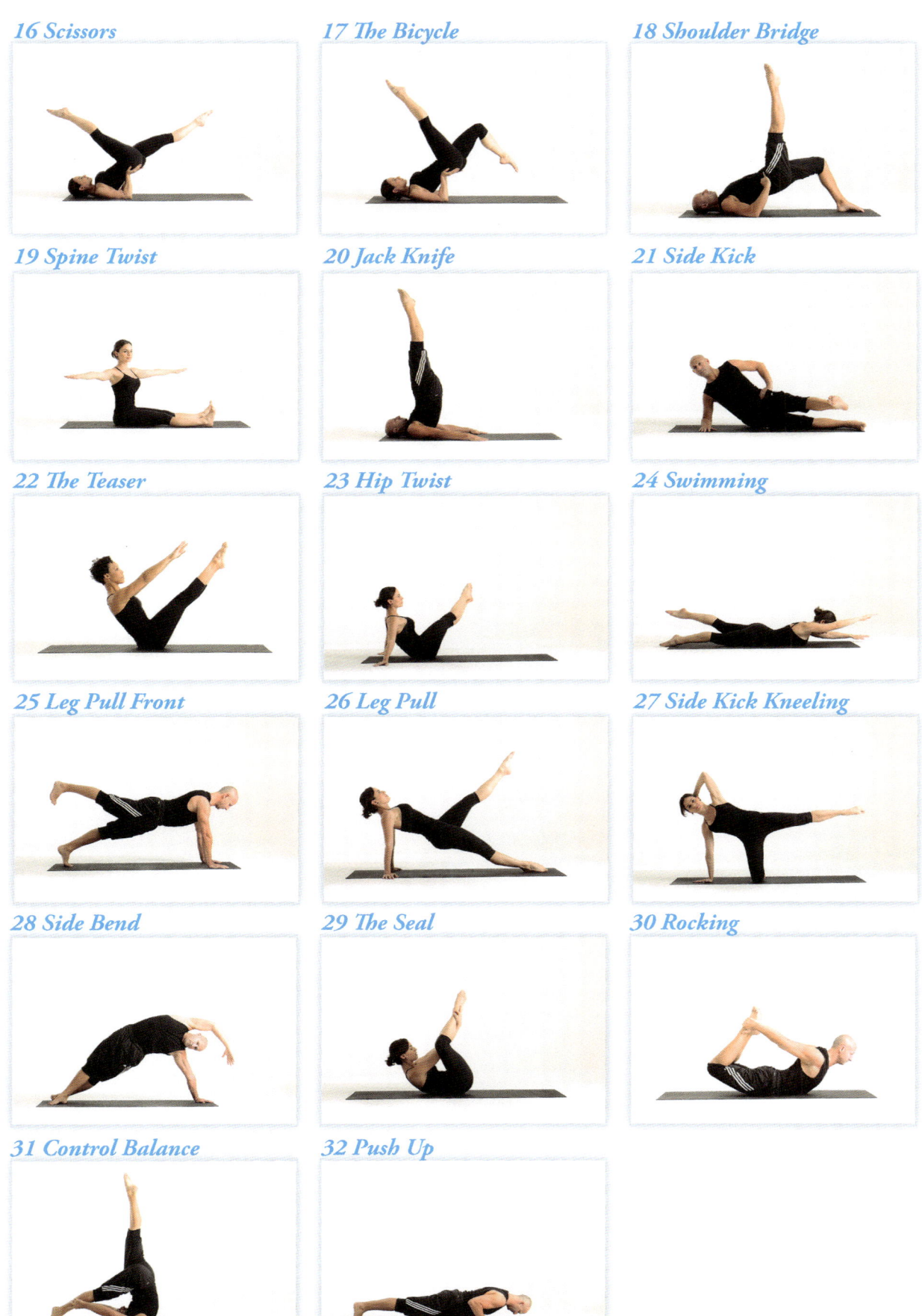

1 The Hundred

Part A – Classical exercises

BACKGROUND

The Hundred is an exercise that doesn't present any major flexibility requirements. Its major challenge is strength in the abdominal and hip flexor muscles and cervical flexors, as well as pectoralis major and minor and latisimuss dorsi. Of course we all require strength in these regions, but repeated performance of the Hundred may reinforce the increasingly common, forward "desk sitting" type of posture. As a consequence, we recommend mostly counterposes; that is, stretching of the major muscles used in the exercise to prevent their adaptive shortening. As we proceed through the book, we will provide both counterposes and stretches that facilitate your ability to perform the classical exercises more safely and correctly.

Major joints and muscles

The ankle is in plantar flexion with a pointed foot. To facilitate this position, try any of the stretches from the extensors and dorsiflexors group in **Chapter 1** for the anterior muscles of the lower leg. An example would be **stretch 5**. Refer to any of the flexors stretches in **Chapter 1** to counteract and stretch the muscles involved, particularly the gastrocnemius. An example would be **stretch 3**.

The hip is in flexion. Refer to the combination quadriceps/hip flexor stretches in **Chapter 3**, in particular **stretch 25, the Floor Godzilla**, for counterposes. The quads and hip flexors work strongly to maintain the extended knee and flexed hip position, so including them in the counterpose is important.

The spine. The entire spine is in flexion. Refer to **Chapter 6** stretches in the extension category for the thoracic and lumbar counterposes. Extending the spine will counteract the shortening of involved muscles like the rectus abdominus, pectoralis major and the like. **Stretch 41, the BOSU Back Bend**, is a nice one to start with. The cervical spine or neck is also in flexion. Refer to **stretch 70 Neck Extension** as the counterpose.

The shoulder is held in internal rotation in the Hundred. Recommended counterposes are **stretches 53 for the latsissimus dorsi, 54 for pectoralis major** and **59 for the internal rotator cuff muscles**.

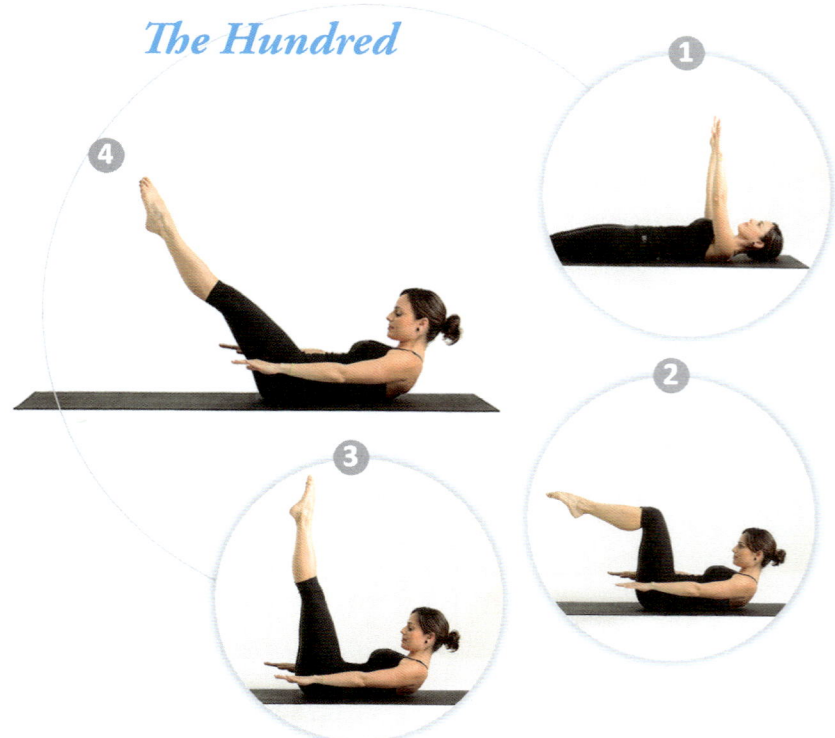

The Hundred

2 The Roll Up

**Part A
Classical exercises**

BACKGROUND

Performing the Roll Up requires significant flexibility in a range of joints and muscles. The final position resembles what in yoga is called the "posterior stretch", because the entire chain of muscles on the posterior side of the body is stretched. (The goal of the Roll Up is supported flexion, whereas the goal of the posterior stretch is maximum flexion.) You may need to practise all of the single joint stretches for several months before you are comfortable in the final position. The Roll Up also uses considerable hip flexor recruitment, so consider inserting a regular hip flexor stretch into your routine if you practise the Roll Up often.

Major joints and muscles

The ankle is dorsi flexed in the Roll Up, requiring flexibility in the calf muscles. Any stretch from the flexors group in **Chapter 1** will assist with this. Try **stretch 1** if unsure.

The knee is in extension, with the pelvis tilted anteriorly during the difficult phases of this exercise. To accomplish this, the hamstrings, gluteus maximus and adductor longus all require significant flexibility. **Stretch 13** will pinpoint all of these accurately.

The Spine is flexed strongly. Try dividing the spine into portions, with flexion stretches for the lumbar and thoracic regions. Try **stretch 37** from Chapter 6 and **Neck Flexion stretch 66** from Chapter 8 first.

When they feel more comfortable, you can demand more from your spine by continuing with the flexion stretches from **Chapter 6** for the entire spine with the neck more strongly included. An example would be **stretch number 40**. Until you can lie supine and flex your hip to 90° with your leg straight, the Roll Up may place strong shearing forces on the joints of the lumbar spine. Thus it should be attempted with great caution.

Our favourite **counterpose** for the Roll Up is **stretch 41, the BOSU Back Bend**. It relieves the spine and neck, as well as the arm and chest muscles like pectoralis major and lats, which work during the exercise.

The Roll Up

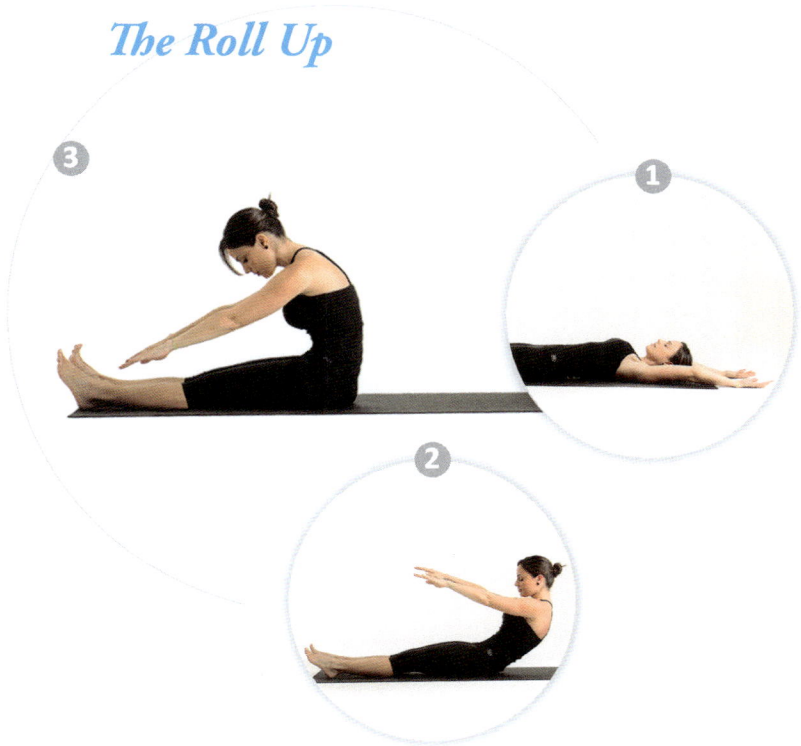

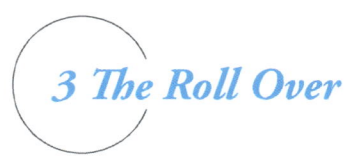

3 The Roll Over

**Part A
Classical exercises**

BACKGROUND

The Roll Over is similar to the Roll Up in its flexibility requirements, the major difference being that the weight of the trunk and legs is atop the neck; whereas, in the Roll Up, the weight of the neck and trunk sit more safely atop the legs. As well as flexibility in the calves, hamstrings and spine, you need almost 90 degrees of flexion in the lower joints of the neck to achieve this exercise. For some this is not achievable, and for others it is not advised. The section on tension and compression will explain the reasons. Check with your teacher before attempting this manoeuvre. The position in photographs 3 and 4 is similar to the "plough pose" in yoga. In the recent book titled *The Science of Yoga: the Risks and the Rewards*, William Broad chronicles several occasions during which stroke has occurred in this position, so practise with a teacher and using caution.

Major joints and muscles

The knee is in extension during the most challenging phases of this exercise, and the pelvis/femur at between 90 to 100 degrees of hip flexion. The posterior thigh and hip muscles need stretching to faciliate this. Practise **stretch 4, the One-Leg Dog Pose**, which reproduces the hip angle perfectly.

The spine is flexed strongly with particular emphasis on the neck. First, practise the **Neck Flexion stretch 66** from Chapter 9. If it is comfortable, then practise **Spinal Flexion stretch 40**.

The shoulders are slightly retracted and the forearm is pronated. For safety, this retraction is critical, so that the weight of the body is distributed across the shoulder blades. For pronation try **stretch 64**. To further facilitate the shoulder retraction, try the **pectoralis minor and anterior deltoid stretch 57**. Complete **stretch 56** for the biceps brachi from Chapter 7 too.

A **counterpose** for the middle trapezius and rhomboids that work hard to stabilise the shoulder girdle is the **Cat stretch, number 39**. For the spine, try the **Cobra stretch 42**.

The Roll Over

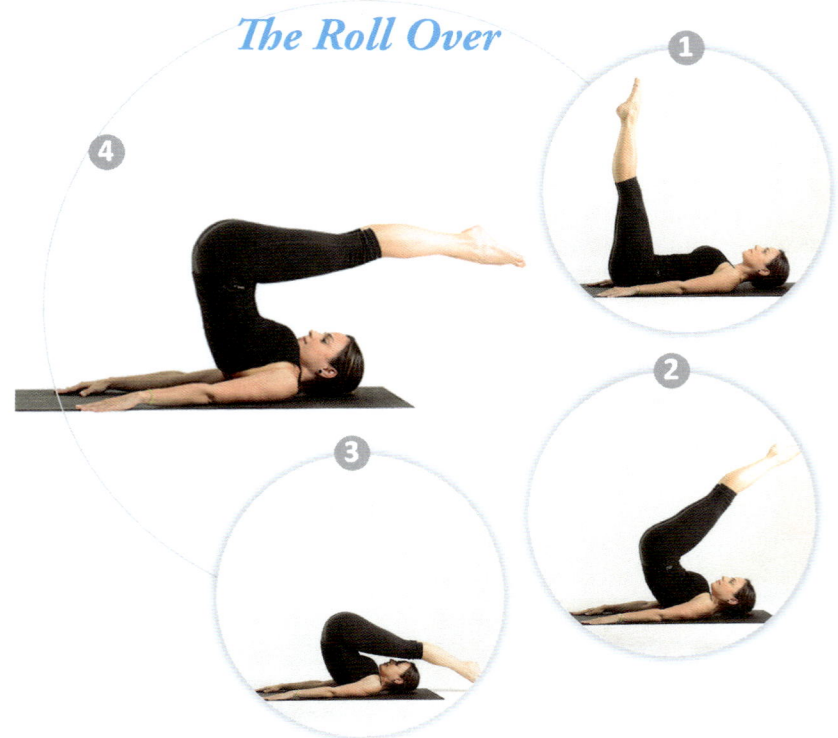

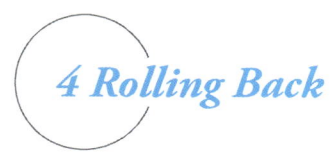
4 Rolling Back

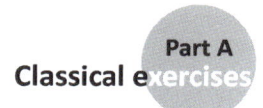
Part A
Classical exercises

BACKGROUND

In Rolling Back the body is held stable in a tight position of knee, hip and trunk flexion. The required flexibility is not demanding, but stretching the quadriceps and gluteus maximus will assist in reaching the position comfortably. Like the Hundred, the posture of Rolling Back is too often maintained in daily life. Because of this, we recommend some counterposes after this exercise.

Major joints and muscles

The hip is also strongly flexed, but because the knees are bent the hamstrings are not under stretch. Rather, it is the gluteus maximus and adductor magnus that need more flexibility here. In particular try **stretch 14 Hamstring Glute Partner** from Chapter 2 for a precise replica of the demands of the Rolling Back.

The spine is strongly flexed but not under as much load as in other mat exercises.

Try any of your favourite stretches from the flexion section of **Chapter 6** in preparation for the Rolling Back.

For **counterposes** we recommend the **Kneeling Hip Flexors, stretch 22**. To counterbalance the flexion of the neck and spine, try the **BOSU Back Bend, stretch 41**. More advanced students with healthy spines can try the **Cobra, stretch 42**.

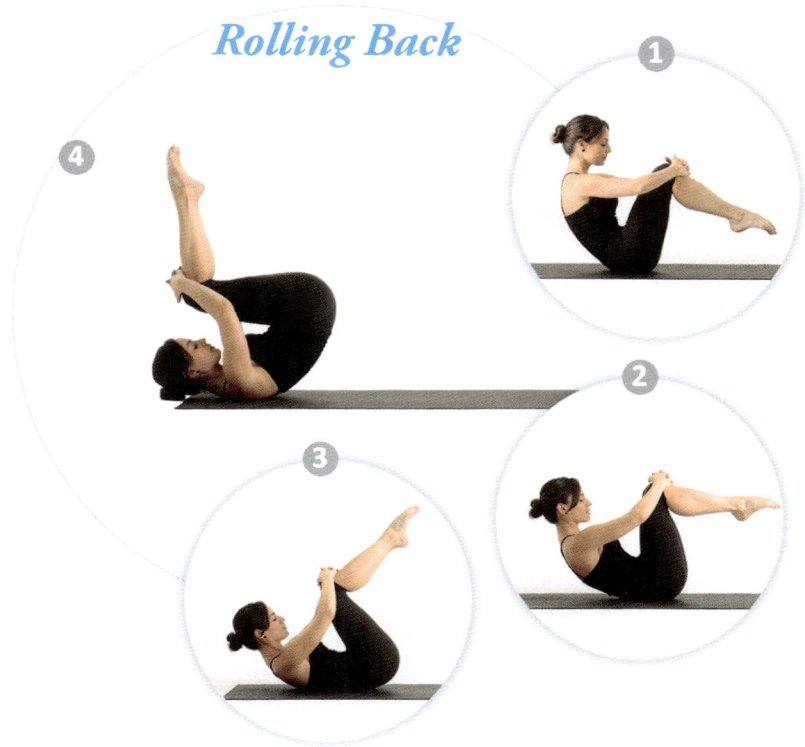

5 One Leg Circle

Part A
Classical exercises

BACKGROUND

Circles performed in both directions require what is known as circumduction at the hip: a combination of flexion, abduction, extension and adduction in one interrelated functional movement. Modern interpretations of the exercise require that the pelvis be kept stable. This makes the flexibility required for its performance even greater, as tension in any of the muscles around the pelvis and hip will cause pelvic movement. Therefore you have two choices: perform the circumduction within a limited range, or develop your flexibility for greater range of movement in the exercise and greater benefit for your hip muscles and joints. Here we'll go with the latter.

Major joints and muscles

The hip is in various combinations of flexion, abduction, adduction and, technically, a movement called extension; although during the exercise the leg never actually moves into an extended position relative to the pelvis.

Flexion of the hip requires length in the hamstrings, adductor magnus and gluteus maximus. Adduction of the hip in the One Leg Circle requires flexibility in the abductors; in particular, the gluteus medius and minimus, TFL and piriformis muscles. **Stretch 15 the Hamstring** replicates all these movement requirements perfectly.

Abduction of the hip requires length in the adductor muscles. There are several of these, and each is stretched in **Chapter Five** with more or less emphasis depending on the precise angle of the leg. For maximum success in this exercise try Chapter Five, stretches **numbers 35** and **36**.

Counterpose: You will notice that your hip flexors work very strongly during this exercise so deserve a good long stretch on its completion. **Stretch 21** will relax both your one and two-joint hip flexors.

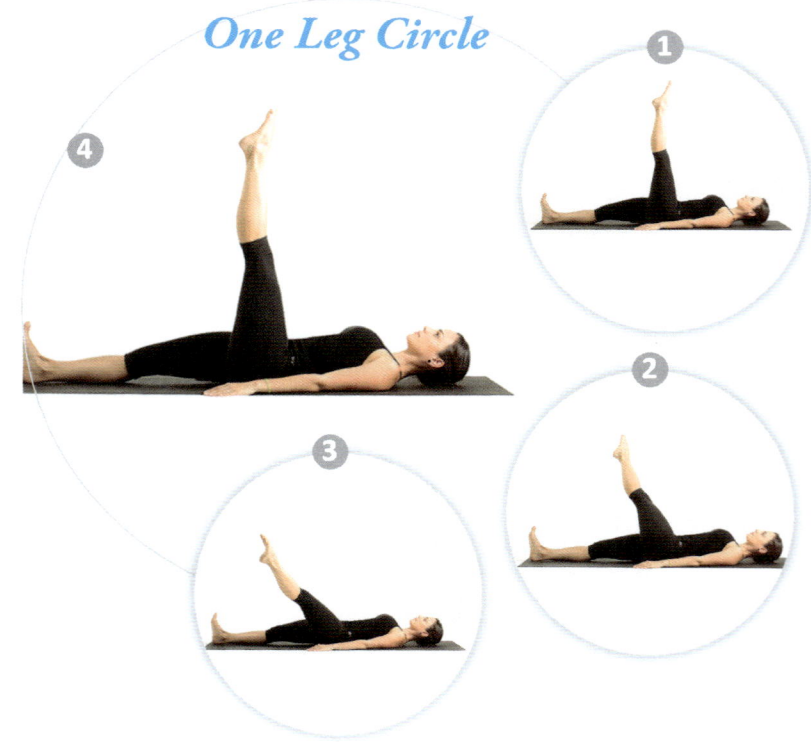

One Leg Circle

6 One Leg Stretch

Part A — Classical exercises

BACKGROUND

Despite its name, the One Leg Stretch is primarily a strength exercise. The major muscles strengthened include the hip flexors and quadriceps, abdominal group and the chest and anterior neck musculature. Tightness in the abdominal wall, in particular the rectus abdominals, can lead to a flexed forward posture as well as inhibition of the deeper and more important abdominal muscles. To combat this, we recommend a series of counterposes to complement this exercise, rewarding and relaxing the major muscles and joints involved in the effort.

Major joints and muscles

The ankle is in plantar flexion during the One Leg Stretch. Try any of the calf stretches from **Chapter One** to counterbalance this tension. To facilitate plantar flexion try **stretch 5**.

The knee both flexes and extends during this exercise. Any of the work from **Chapter Three** will provide wonderful relaxation for the hip flexor and quadriceps muscles groups. **Stretch 21** is the most efficient, stretching both groups in the one exercise. For the hip extensors try **stretch 19**.

The Spine remains strongly flexed during the single leg stretch.

Try a strong abdominal stretch from **Chapter Six** to lengthen the abdominal muscles as a counterpose. The seated back bend over the BOSU ball, **stretch 41**, is a lovely one to begin with. This will also stretch the anterior neck muscles that are isometrically contracted throughout the exercise.

The shoulder, called the glenohumeral joint, is flexed and adducted during the One Leg Stretch. The pectoralis major works hard during this movement (with countless others assisting), so reward it with a stretch. Try the **pec stretch, number 55**, from Chapter Seven as the counterpose.

One Leg Stretch

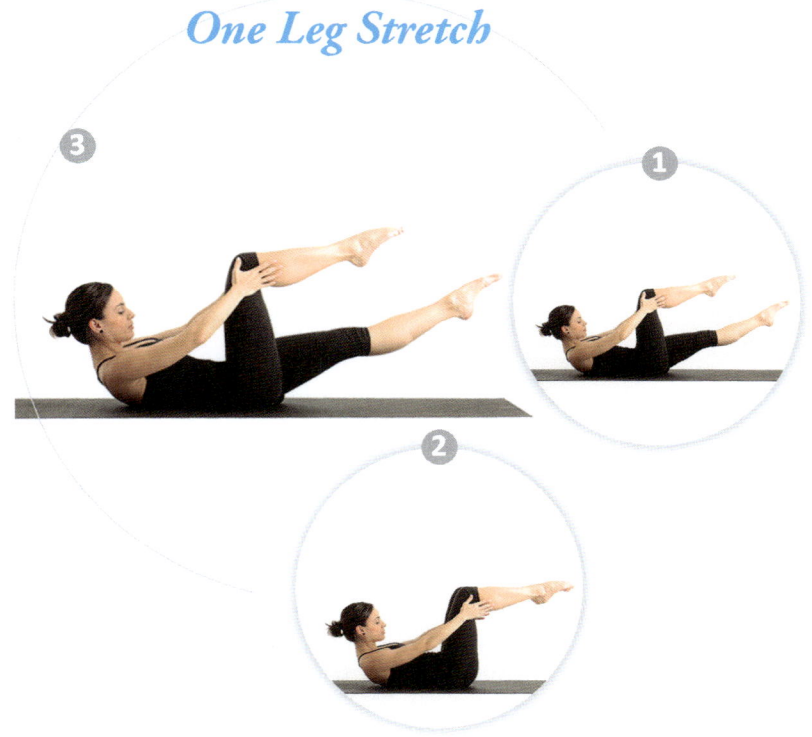

7 Double Leg Stretch

Part A — Classical exercises

BACKGROUND

Like the One Leg Stretch, the Double Leg Stretch demands strength rather than flexibility for its performance. The strength demands are increased because both legs are extended from the body at the same time. Knee, hip and spine flexion is required and, as with the One Leg Stretch, counterposes are recommended. For these, please follow all recommendations for the One Leg Stretch.

Major joints and muscles

The hip is strongly flexed. This requires good range of movement through the joint as well as flexibility in the gluteus maximus, hamstrings and adductor longus. **Stretch 14 Hamstring** is a terrific compound stretch for these muscles. "Compound" in this context means it will target all three muscles at the same time. Any stretch from **Chapters Four** and **Five** will also supplement this one.

The Spine requires flexion throughout. Try **stretch 39 the Cat** as it replicates this movement closely.

Counterposes. All the anterior muscles of the body, including abdominals, hip and neck flexors, work hard during this exercise. **Stretch 41 the BOSU Back Bend** will provide an efficient counterpose.

The hip flexors may tire and ache after this exercise, so we also recommend **stretch 22 Kneeling Hip Flexor**.

In addition, try **stretch 3 Lying Calf with Strap**, as pointing the foot repeatedly may shorten the gastrocnemius and others.

Double Leg Stretch

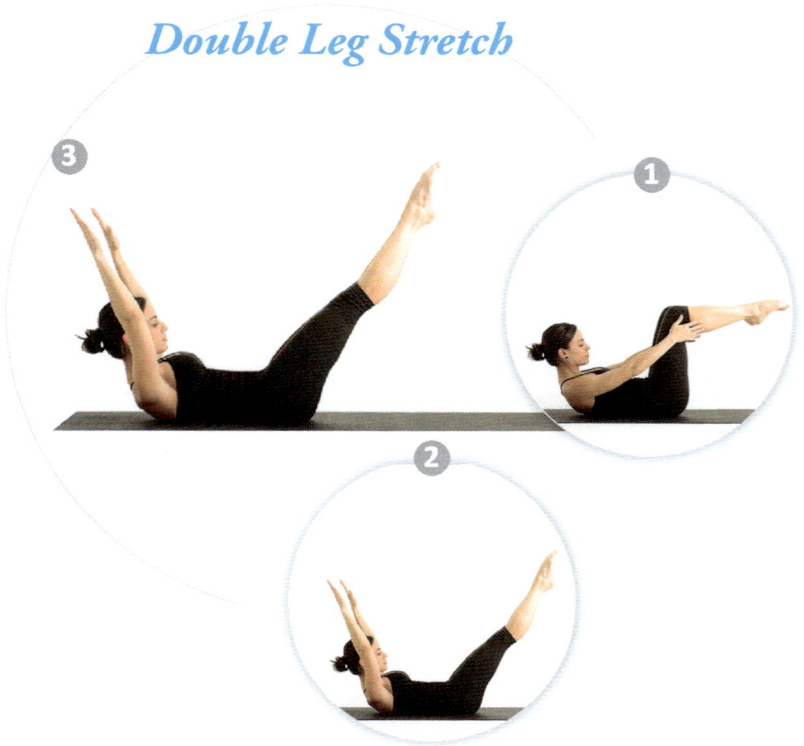

8 Spine Stretch

**Part A
Classical exercises**

BACKGROUND

The Spine Stretch is another flexion-based movement. It is similar to the Roll Up but requires less abdominal work. For stabilisation, the initial position requires work in the erector spinae, hip flexors, abdominal and quadratus lumborum muscles, so counterposes for these groups will be recommended. In the final position, significant flexibility is required in the entire posterior spine, calves, hamstrings and gluteus maximus. The latissimus dorsi and long head of triceps and rhomboids in particular also require a moderate amount of extensibility to enable you to reach between the feet. We will look at some stretches for these also.

Major joints and muscles

The ankles are kept in dorsi flexion throughout the exercise, requiring length in the calf muscles. Start with one of the sitting exercises for the calves, perhaps with your foot in a strap, **stretch 3**.

The knee is in extension, with the pelvis tilted anteriorly. Consequently, you need to stretch the hamstring group and gluteus maximus. Try **stretch 12 the Foam Roller**, which reproduces the demands of the exercise precisely.

The spine is held in strong flexion, so try any of the positions in the flexion section in **Chapter Six**. **Stretch 37** mimics the position closely. In addition, try some of the seated flexion stretches for the neck from **Chapter Nine**, such as **stretch 66**.

The shoulder is in flexion, and the movement of reaching toward the feet requires adequate length in the lats and the long head of the triceps. For the lats, go to **stretch 53** in particular. For the long head of triceps, attempt **stretch 58** from Chapter Seven. For the rhomboids, **stretch 48 Pull and Push** is the best. This enables the protraction of the scapula.

Counterposes for the hip flexors can be found in **Chapter Three**. The hip flexors pull the trunk toward the leg.

For the spine and abdominals, try one of the versions of the **Cobra stretch, number 42**.

Spine Stretch

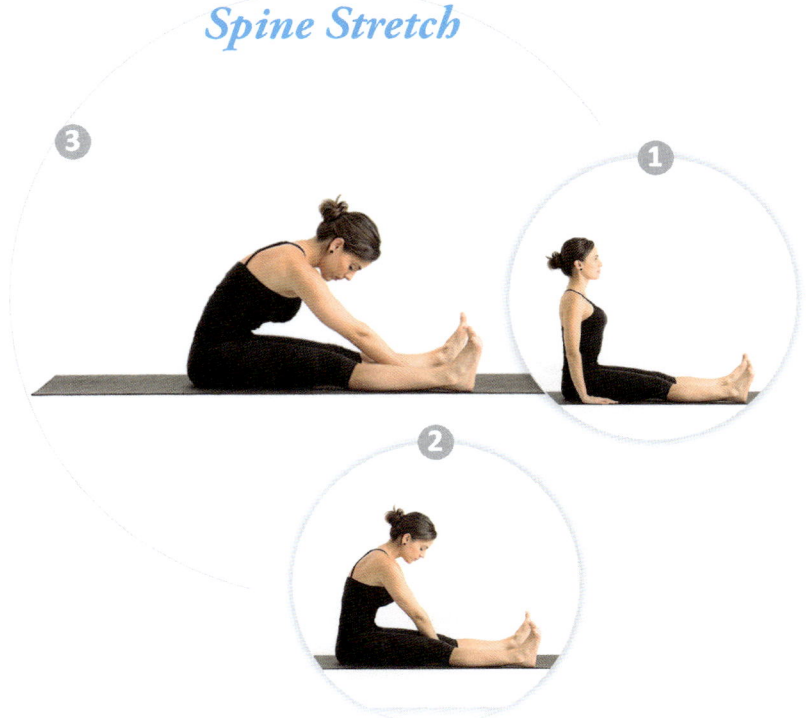

9 Rocker with Open legs

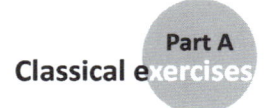

**Part A
Classical exercises**

BACKGROUND

Apart from the obvious strength, balance and coordination challenges of this exercise, a good degree of abduction in the legs is required, as well as flexion of the entire trunk. The hip flexors work very hard too in maintaining the flexed hip position throughout the exercise. A couterpose that elongates the hip flexors is a good idea when you finish your practice.

Major joints and muscles

The hips are abducted, requiring flexibility in the adductor muscle group. Any of the work in **Chapter Five** will provide good preparation and long-term improvement. In addition, the medial hamstrings in particular need stretching for this exercise. Try **stretch 33** in Chapter Five, Kneeling Short Long. This exercise will stretch both adductors and medial hamstrings.

The spine is flexed throughout the Rocker. Try your favourite flexion stretch from **Chapter Six** to prepare for this. Select a neck flexion stretch from **Chapter nine** for the neck. An example would be **stretch 66**.

Beware of excessive flexion of the cervical spine during this movement, particularly with the weight of the body bearing down on the neck. Check with your teacher as to the suitability of the exercise and note the position in image 4 below; you should not roll back further than onto the shoulders.

Counterposes for the hip flexors can be selected from **Chapter Three**. In addition, you can do the backbend over the BOSU ball to bend your spine in the other direction, **stretch 41**.

Rocker with Open Legs

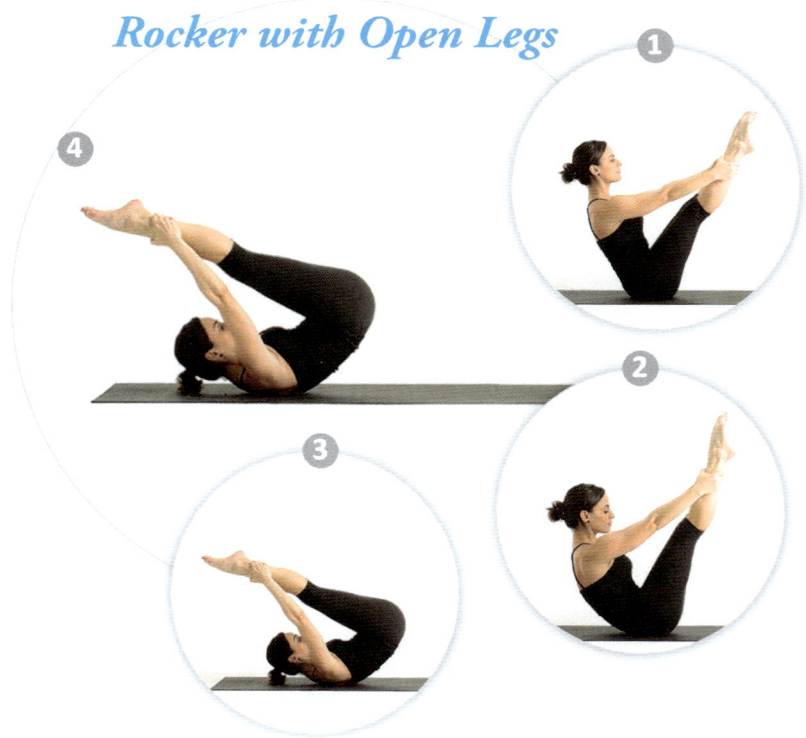

10 The Cork Screw

Part A
Classical exercises

BACKGROUND

The cork screw requires a flexed lumbar spine, strong hip flexor contraction and considerable work from the lats and erector spinae to stabilise the upper body and shoulders onto the mat. If they are tight, the pectoralis minor and biceps brachi will prevent the shoulder blades from lying flat on the mat. Please observe where your shoulders lie when lying passively in preparation for this exercise. If the front of the shoulders tends to sit up from the mat, try the recommendations below. The shoulders are also required to be in internal rotation. To facilitate this position try the recommendations below.

Major joints and muscles

The hips are in flexion. Refer to any of the straight leg hamstring stretches to facilitate this position. An example is **stretch 16**.

The spine is in flexion in the lumbar region, so in preparation practise **stretch 38 the Dangler** from Chapter Six.

The shoulders should lie flat on the mat. Try **stretch 57** for the pectoralis minor and biceps brachi **stretch 56** to enable this position.

In addition, stretch the external rotator cuff muscles with **stretch 60** to facilitate this position.

Counterposes for the spine can include any of the flexion exercises from **Chapter 6**. In addition, try **42 the Cobra** for some lumber extension.

A relaxing counter pose for the latissimus dorsi and trunk muscles is **stretch 53**.

A **counterpose** for the shoulders is the **internal rotator cuff stretch 61**.

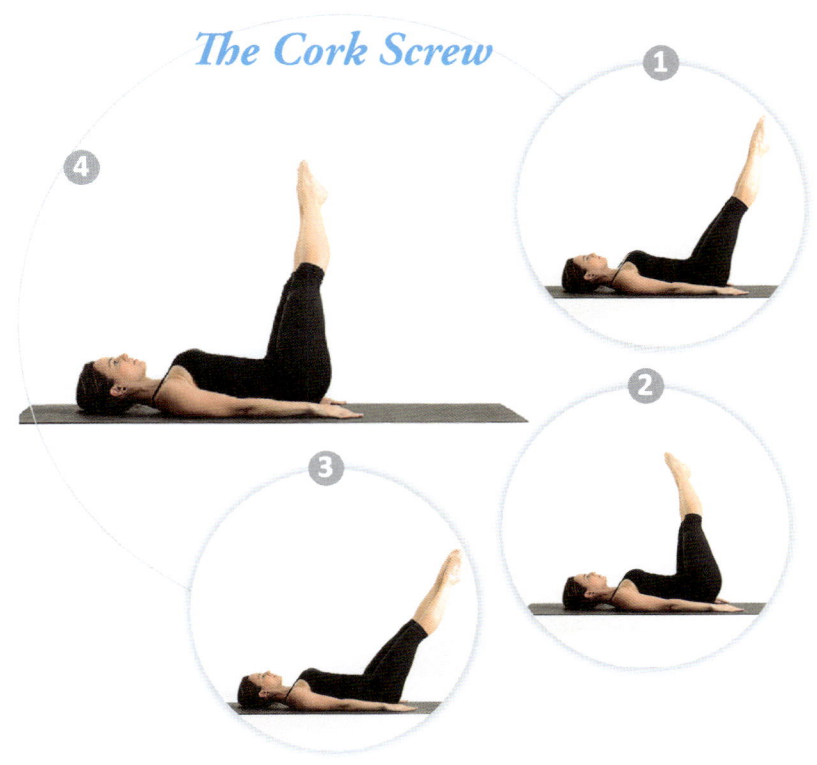

The Cork Screw

11 The Saw

Part A Classical exercises

BACKGROUND

The Saw involves a combination of spinal rotation and flexion. Throughout the exercise the legs are abducted and the knees extended. To enable you to sit straight, substantial flexibility in the adductors and hamstrings is required. Correct performance of this seemingly simple exercise requires flexibility at a range of joints and muscles in the body, as described below.

Major joints and muscles

The ankle is in dorsi flexion. Practise **stretch 2 Standing Calf** first, then progress to stronger versions like **stretch 4 the One Leg Dog Pose**.

The knees are extended. In order to sit up in this position, practise a straight-leg hamstring stretch from Chapter Two, **stretch 16**.

The hips are abducted, requiring good flexibility in the adductor muscles. Try any of the seated or lying straight leg stretches in **Chapter Five** in preparation. **Stretch number 34** is perfect.

The spine is both rotated and flexed. An exercise that combines both movements without the added difficulty of extended legs is **stretch 48 Pull and Push** in Chapter Six.

In addition, you can practise rotation alone with **seated rotation stretch 45** in Chapter Six. A spinal flexion stretch from **Chapter Six** will also facilitate the final position in the Saw. Try **the Accelerator, stretch 37**.

Counterposes for the Saw are **stretch 38 the Dangler** (the erector spinae work hard in the Saw, so reward them with a good dangle!), while to reverse the lumber flexion try **42 the Cobra**. You may also feel an ache in the hip flexors, particularly if your hamstrings are tight, because the hip flexor muscles must work against them to sit you up straight. Try **stretch number 22** as an antidote.

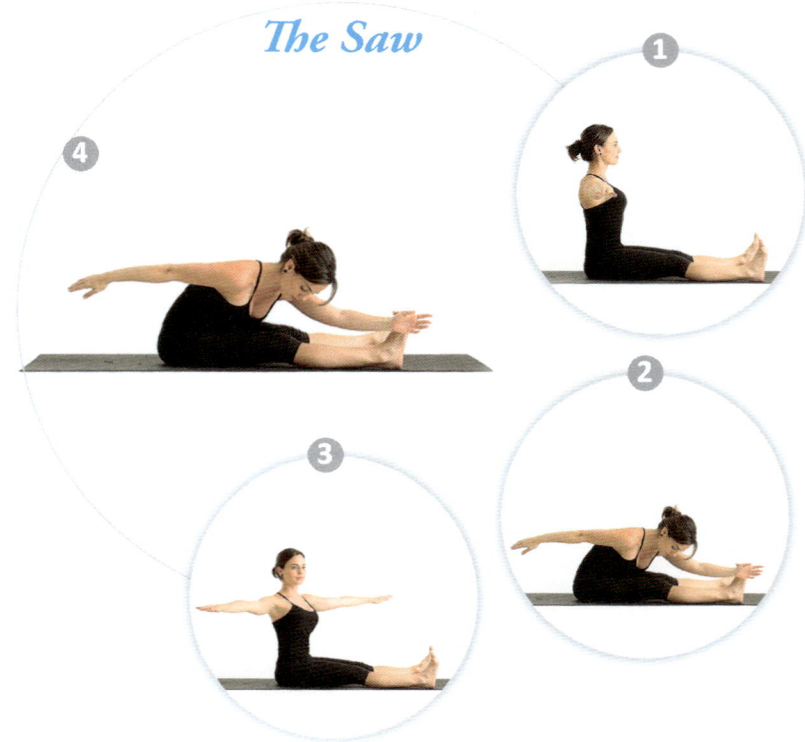

The Saw

12 Swan Dive

Part A
Classical exercises

BACKGROUND

In this modified version of the original, the thoracic and lumber spine is extended, the chest is open, and the hips are extended. In addition, the feet are strongly pointed or planter flexed, requiring flexibility in the anterior muscles of the lower leg. If you are particularly stiff, you may want to consider attempting only the first and second positions for several months while practising the stretches. If your lower back is uncomfortable in this extended position, check with your teacher for advice.

Major joints and muscles

The ankle is strongly pointed or plantar flexed. This requires strength in the calves, but also adequate length in the anterior muscles of the lower leg. Try **stretch 21** in preparation; although it is in **Chapter 3**, it definitely stretches the lower leg.

The hips are extended in the final pose, strengthening the glutes but also demanding flexibility in their opposing muscles, the hip flexors. Try any of the hip flexor stretches from **Chapter Three** to enable this movement.

The Spine is in significant extension during the last phases of Swan Dive, so try some supported extension exercises before you attempt this one.

The back extension over the **BOSU ball, stretch 41**, is a safe one to try and can be found in **Chapter Six**. If you are comfortable with this, try **42 the Cobra** pose with arms wide first and proceed to the stronger versions from there.

The chest is not a joint in itself, but requires expansion during the Swan Dive. The BOSU back extension will assist with this, but length in the pectoral muscles, both major and minor, should also be attended to. Try **stretch 54** in Chapter 7.

To flex the spine, a lovely counterpose for this exercise is **the Dangler, stretch number 38**.

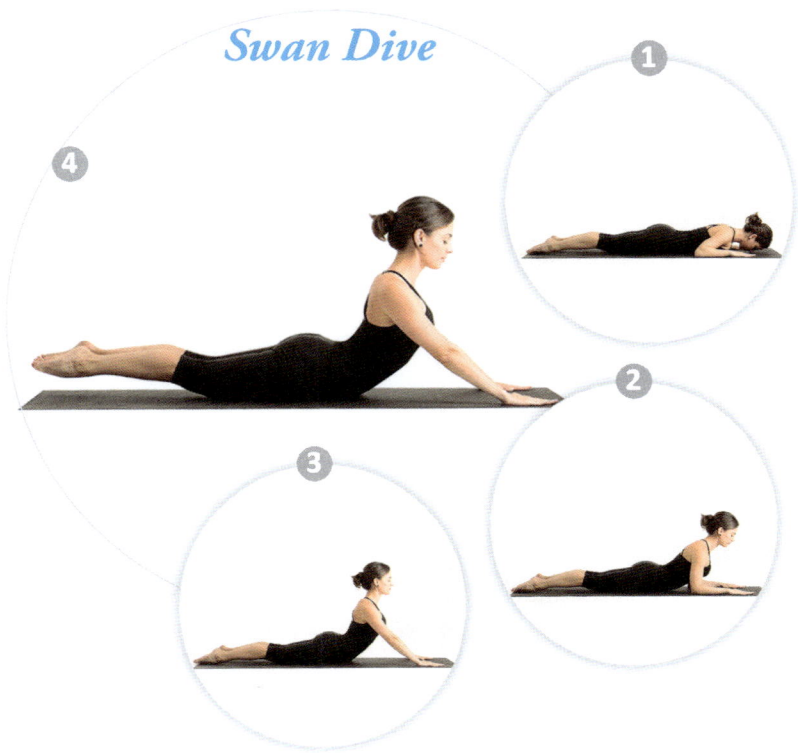

13 One Leg Kick

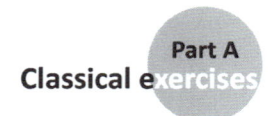
Part A
Classical exercises

BACKGROUND

The One Leg Kick is an exercise that requires coordination and control. As the knee bends, the hamstrings work – then suddenly the quadriceps becomes active to curtail the movement. The spine is in a moderate amount of extension throughout. When the knee is flexed, the quadriceps must lengthen to allow the movement and limit the pull of the rectus femoris on the lumbar spine and pelvis.

Major joints and muscles

The spine, particularly the lumber spine, is held in extension. Try any of the supported back bends from **Chapter Six** to facilitate this position. The supported position will offer less compressive load on the spine and its structures than in the One Leg Kick. **The hip flexors**, if they are tight, will make the extended lumbar position less comfortable. Stretch them first using partner **stretch 23** to lengthen the one and two-joint hip flexors.

The knee is flexed. Try one of the quadriceps stretches from **Chapter Three** to facilitate this. If you have just performed **stretch 23**, you do not need to do a second one.

A **counterpose** for the hamstrings and lower back would be sensible. Try **stretch 12 the Foam Roller Hamstring**. This is an excellent stretch that will lengthen the lumbar spine hamstrings and calves simultaneously.

One Leg Kick

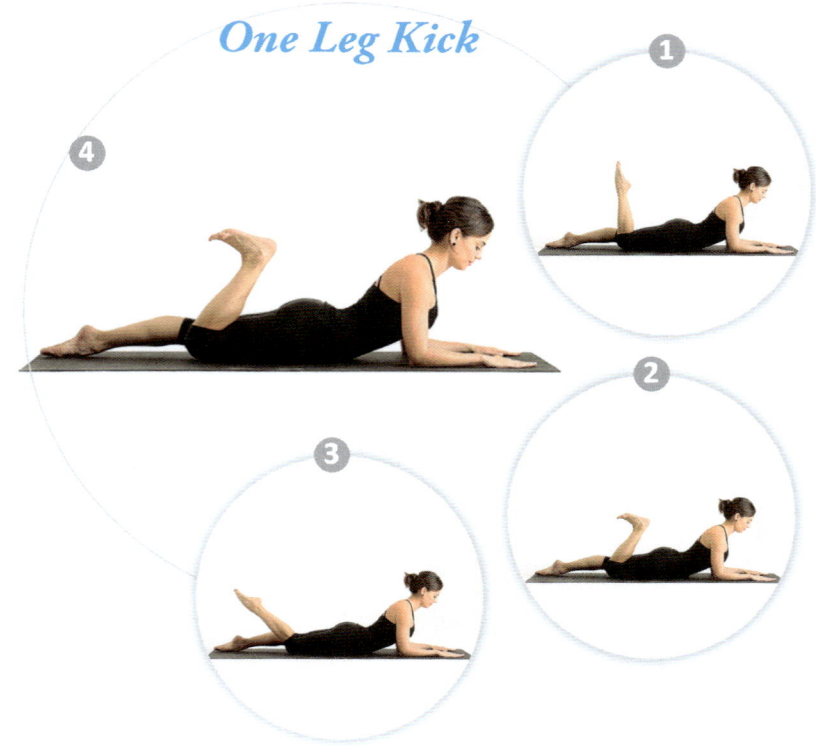

14 Double Leg Kick

Part A — Classical exercises

BACKGROUND

The Double Leg Kick requires some strong hip extension and spine extension as well as significant extension of the shoulder joint. Shoulder extension such as this demands flexibility in the pectoralis minor, biceps brachii and anterior deltoid muscles. The hip flexor muscles need adequate length to allow the kicking motion. A counterpose should be performed following this exercise due to the compression load on the lumbar joints.

Major joints and muscles

The hip is extended during parts of the Double Leg Kick. To prevent the lumbar spine being too strongly extended during this movement, stretch the rectus femoris and the one-joint hip flexors. **Stretch 25 the Godzilla** will serve well to facilitate the required hip extension.

The knee is flexed. As mentioned above, perform the Godzilla to lengthen the quadriceps for this task.

The lumbar spine can be extended using any of the work in the extension section in **Chapter Six**. **The Cobra, stretch 42**, mimics this position closely.

The shoulder joint is in strong extension. Try stretching the pectoralis minor with **stretch 57** from Chapter Seven, following with **stretch 56 Lying Bicep**. This stretch will also take care of your anterior deltoid. If you are stiff, it may take several months of work before you are able to extend your arms and shoulders as pictured. For the neck rotation try **stretch 69**.

Counterpose using the **Accelerator stretch 37** in the spinal flexion section from **Chapter Six**. This is a lovely counterpose for the spine and middle trapezius muscles in particular.

The Double Leg Kick

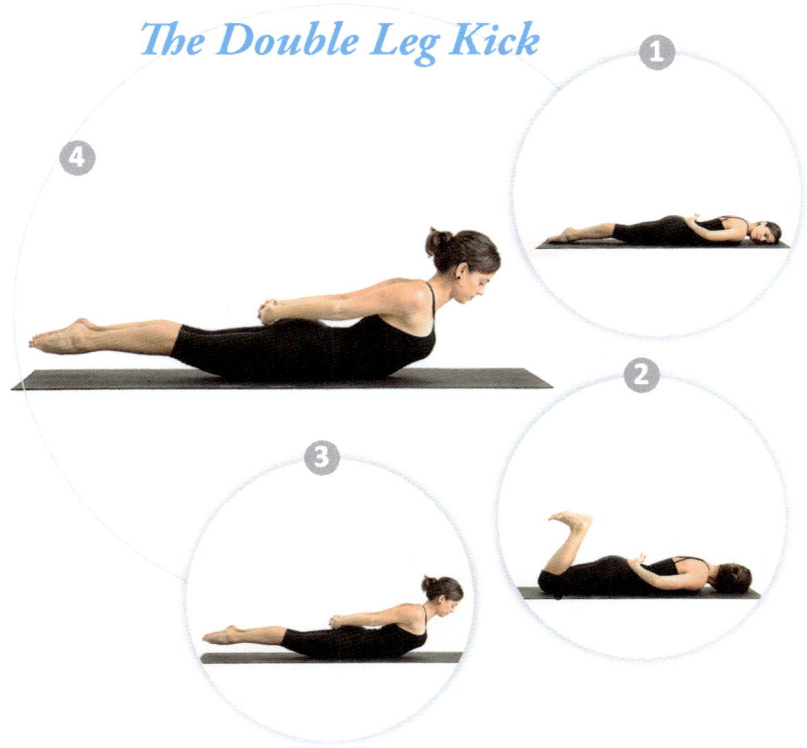

15 Neck Pull

Part A
Classical exercises

BACKGROUND

The essential flexibility requirements of the Neck Pull are calf and hamstring length, as well as spinal flexion. The hip flexors and abdominal muscles work hard during this exercise to bend the trunk and pull it toward the legs. Try a counterpose for these areas if you feel tight after this exercise.

Major joints and muscles

The ankle is dorsi flexed. Try one of the seated or lying calf stretches to produce strong dorsi flexion without those antagonistic muscles, the calves, preventing the movement. **Stretch 3** is an example.

The hips are also strongly flexed, as well as the pelvis rotating anteriorly. This requires considerable length in the hamstrings and, secondarily, in the gluteus maximus and adductor magnus. Try **26 the Lunge Pose** from Chapter Three for the gluteal and adductor stretch. Proceed to **Chapter Two** for a strong series of hamstring stretches. **Stretch 16** is appropriate.

If you want to include some spinal flexion in your hamstring stretch try **stretch 13**. Otherwise, break down the Neck Pull further by focusing on the hamstrings separately, then the spine.

The spine is strongly flexed. Try any flexion stretch from **Chapter Six**, as well as **neck flexion stretch 56** from Chapter 9 to facilitate this.

Counterpose. If you feel like a counterpose to the Neck Pull, select any of the stretches from the spinal extension in **Chapter Six** to reverse the movement. Take your pick.

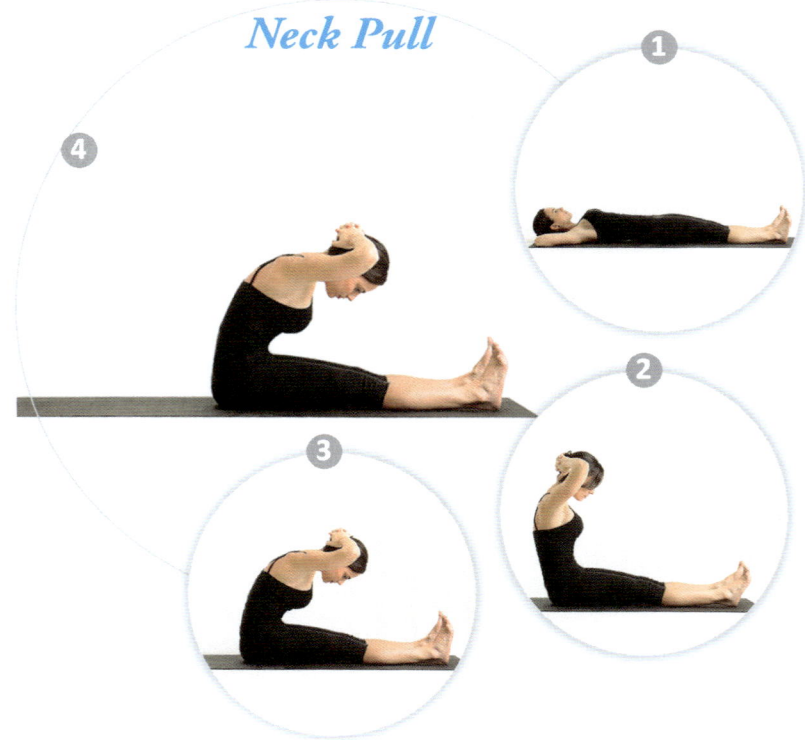

Neck Pull

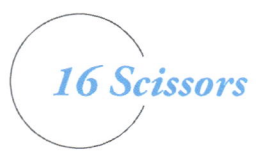

16 Scissors

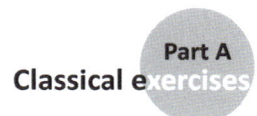

**Part A
Classical exercises**

BACKGROUND

The Scissors require a strong degree of neck flexion, which must be performed with caution. In addition, the criss-crossing movement of the legs can be accomplished only with good flexibility through the hip joints. Keeping the shoulders on the mat requires strength in some of the scapula retractors like the trapezius and rhomboids, and good flexibility in the pectoralis minor muscles so that the scapula can be retracted.

Major joints and muscles

The hips are both flexed and extended. To stretch the hip flexors so that the hip can be extended, try **stretch 26 the Lunge Pose** in Chapter Three.

The hamstrings are best prepared for this stretch using one of the straight leg hamstring stretches from **Chapter Two**. **Stretch 16** is perfect.

The spine is flexed strongly in the cervical region. Try one of the neck flexion stretches from **Chapter Eight**; for example, **stretch 66**. Proceed with caution because the neck is not always comfortable bearing weight through these joints, particularly if your vertebrae are large or the process long.

Check out the section on tension and compression for further information.

The shoulder/scapula joint requires some retraction. **Stretch 57 Standing Pectoralis Minor** is a perfect replica of this movement. In addition, try **55 Lying Pec Major**. Perform both, and once you have experienced the openness of the chest, your Scissors performance will feel more graceful and fluid.

As a **counterpose** for the wrists, which bear considerable weight during this exercise, try the **wrist extension stretch 62**.

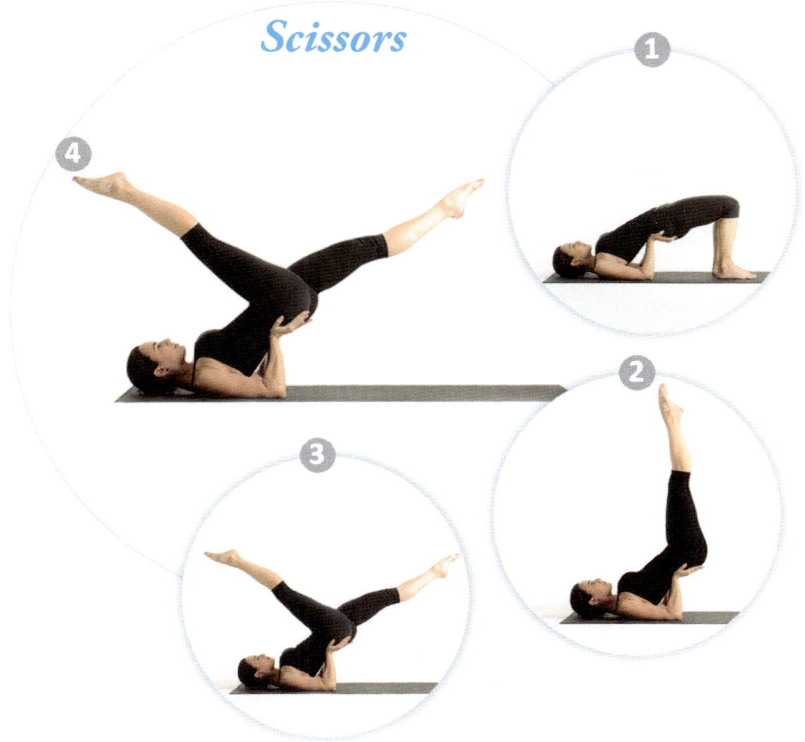

Scissors

17 The Bicycle

**Part A
Classical exercises**

BACKGROUND

The bicycle is similar to the previous exercise, Scissors. The main flexibility requirement is in the neck. Because the knees are bent in the bicycle, the leg muscles are slackened and require less flexibility. As a consequence, we will recommend some counterposes to give them a stretch after you perform the exercise.

Major joints and muscles

The spine is strongly flexed at the neck. Try **neck flexion stretch 66** from Chapter Eight.

The shoulders are retracted. To facilitate this position, try the **pec minor stretch 57** and the **pec major stretch 55**.

Counterposes for the neck and legs are recommended after performing the bicycle. Try **Neck Extension Stretch 70** from Chapter nine to take the head and neck in the opposite direction.

The quadriceps and hip flexors work hard during this exercise. Reward them with some stretching afterwards.

Try the **Lying Quadricep stretch 23**, or, if you are up for it, **25 the Floor Godzilla** and include a partner if you have one.

Although it can be hard to see, the lumbar spine is held in extension in many versions of this stretch. **Stretch numbers 37** to **40** would all be suitable as counterposes to this position.

Stretch 42 Cobra is a multijoint exercise that will stretch your lower back and neck simultaneously, in the opposite direction to the Bicycle.

The **Pull and Push stretch 48** will help relax the middle trapezius and rhomboids, which work strongly to hold the body in position.

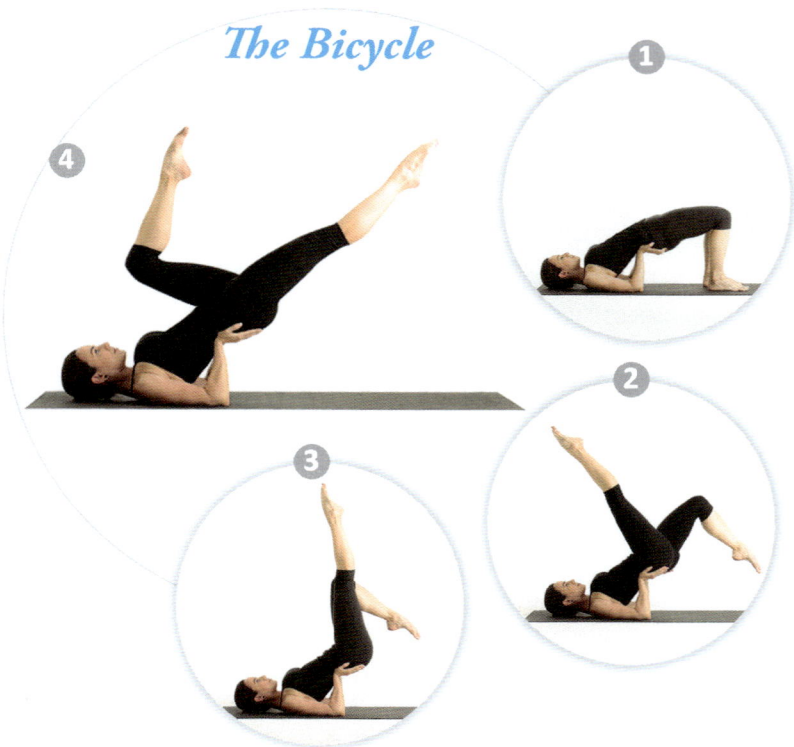

The Bicycle

18 Shoulder Bridge

Part A
Classical exercises

BACKGROUND

The Shoulder Bridge is a demanding exercise strength-wise, while lifting the leg into hip flexion requires considerable flexibility in the hamstrings. The neck is flexed again, so refer to the previous few stretches for advice in this area. In addition, the shoulders are held flat on the mat. This tests the pectoralis minor length and the gluteal muscles work hard to hold the body in the bridge position. The hip flexors must be stretched, as tension in the hip flexors can inhibit the gluteal muscles from activating.

Major joints and muscles

The hip is flexed when the leg is lifted from the floor. To facilitate this position stretch the hamstring strongly with any of the work from **Chapter Two**. Try **stretch 18** for a different approach.

The hip flexors require a degree of flexibility to enable the supporting leg to lift the hip. As described above, relaxing the hip flexors will permit stronger contraction of the gluteals. Try **stretch 20** as a facilitating stretch.

The shoulder joints are protracted, requiring flexibility in the anterior deltoid and pectoral muscles, "pec minor" in particular. Try **stretches 55** and **57**.

Counterpose. The erector spinae work hard during the Shoulder Bridge, so **stretch 39 the Cat** will be a relaxing counterpose.

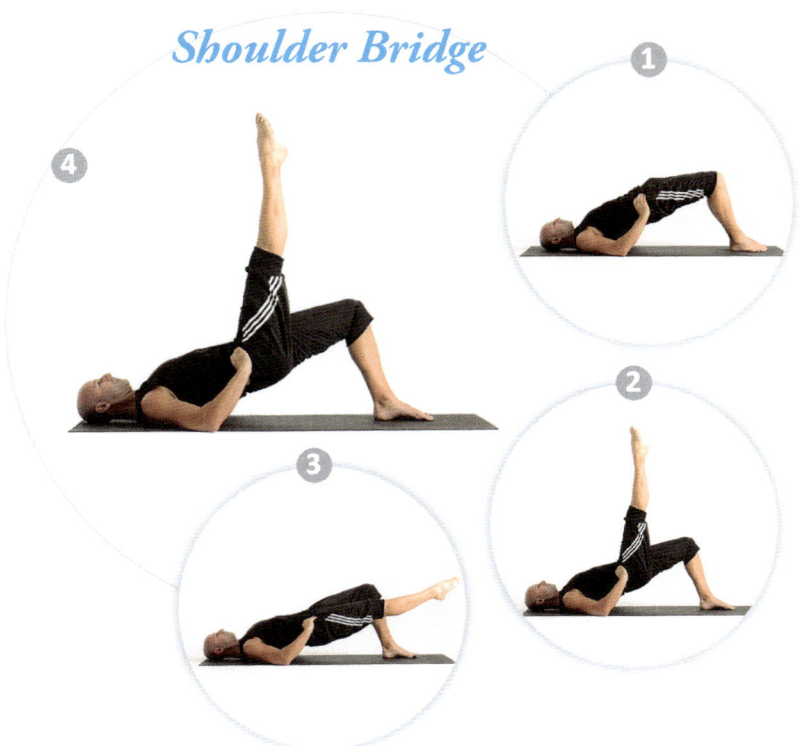

Shoulder Bridge

19 Spine Twist

**Part A
Classical exercises**

BACKGROUND

The spine twist is an elegant exercise requiring the following flexibility requirements: length in the calves, hamstrings and long adductors to enable the sitting position, and the ability of the joints of the thoracic spine and the oblique abdominal muscles to enable rotation of the trunk.

Major joints and muscles

The ankle is dorsi flexed. This requires sufficient calf muscle length. Try any of the calf exercises to prepare for this portion of the exercise. **Stretch 3** is an example.

The knee is extended, requiring significant flexibility in the hamstrings and the long adductors like adductor magnus – particularly to allow the sitting position. Try both versions of **stretch 15**. This is an excellent preparatory stretch for the spine twist because the variations will move the stretch through the entire hamstring and adductor group.

The spine is rotated. Most of the rotation is in the thoracic and cervical joints and their surrounding muscles. To prepare for or facilitate the movement, the most suitable stretch is the **Seated Rotation, stretch 45**. You might add the **neck rotation 69** also.

Counterpose. The erector spinae work hard to maintain the vertical spine throughout this excercise. Try **stretch 39** as a relaxing movement for these muscles.

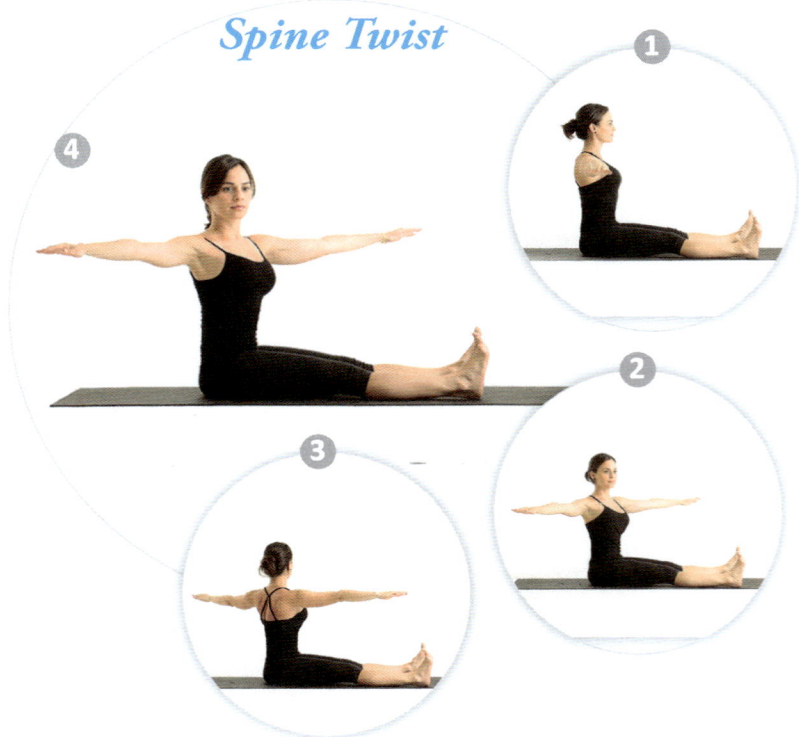

20 Jack Knife

Part A — Classical exercises

BACKGROUND

The Jack Knife requires some spinal and hamstring length in the intermediate positions where the spine and hips are both flexed. In the final position there is significant load on the lower cervical joints, so this position is not for everyone. Consider that there is widespread variation in the bony architecture among the "average" neck, and some will not allow a 90 degree bend. If this applies to you, do not attempt the vertical position, and allow for some hip flexion to counterbalance the fact that your trunk cannot be at 90 degrees to the floor. The shoulders are in extension also, requiring some chest expansion work.

Major joints and muscles

The spine is flexed through its entirety at various points in the exercise, including the very last position if you are able to achieve it. To prepare the thoracic and lumbar spine, try the **Accelerator stretch 37**. The neck must be flexed strongly in preparation, so try **stretch 66** from Chapter Nine. If you are unable to perform considerable neck flexion whilst seated, it would not be a good idea to continue to the Jack Knife.

The hips are also flexed during various stages, so complete some seated hamstring and spinal stretches like **12 the Foam Roller Hamstring** in preparation.

The shoulders are in extension, requiring flexibility in the anterior deltoids, the biceps and the pectoral muscles – in particular, pectoralis minor. A compound stretch of all of these muscles is the **Lying Bicep stretch 56**. Try this movement to prepare your chest for this exercise. Without it, the weight of your body will be experienced further on the neck, and less on the scapula.

Counterpose. Because both the anterior and posterior chain of muscles work hard in the Jack Knife, we recommended the **Cobra stretch 43** and the **Advanced Dangler stretch 40**.

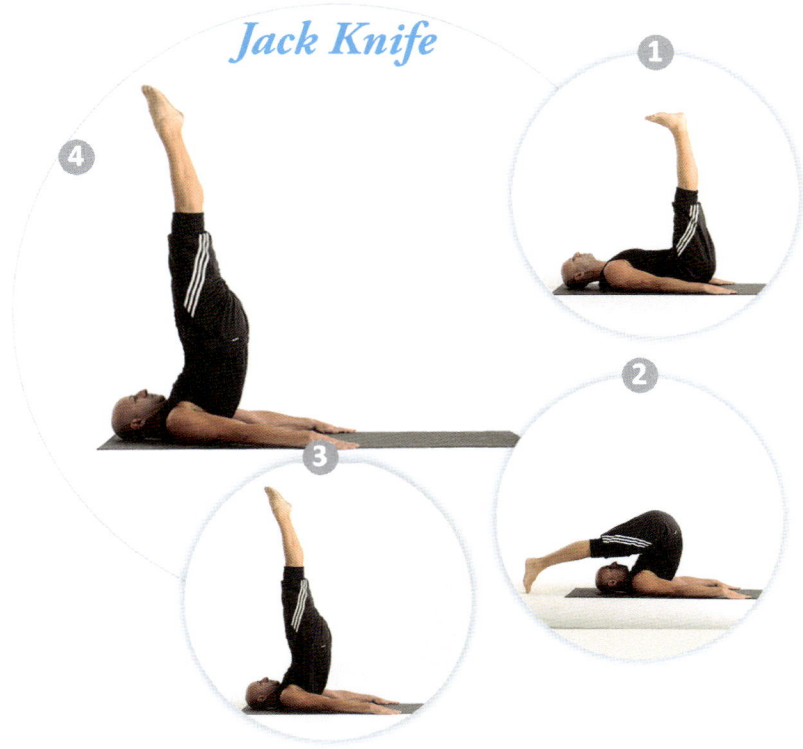

Jack Knife

21 Side Kick

**Part A
Classical exercises**

BACKGROUND

The Side Kick challenges the core muscles of the trunk, and inflexibility in the hamstrings and hip flexors will make the core appear weak, even if it is not. This is because swinging the leg back and forth stretches the hamstrings and hip flexors alternately, pulling strongly on the pelvis and spine and overpowering the ability of the core muscles. Greater flexibility in these muscles will enable far greater stability in the trunk. In the version we have chosen to include, the body is held on the elbow and shoulder. We will try a counterpose for some of the muscles doing the work around these joints too.

Major joints and muscles

The hips require flexion and extension capabilities. Try any of the exercises in **Chapter Two** for the hamstrings and **Chapter Three** for hip flexors to facilitate these movements.

The shoulder is held at roughly 90 degrees to the trunk, working the lats, deltoids and abdominal muscles strongly. In particular, the quadratus lumborum (QL) will work to support the trunk.

Try **stretch 53** for the latissimus dorsi first. Proceed to the **rotator cuff stretches 59** and **60**, and then to the **Foam Roller Mermaid stretch 49** for the QL. The abductor muscles of the bottom leg and hip will also work strongly to brace the pelvis, so try the **seated hip stretch 27** to prevent soreness and stiffness.

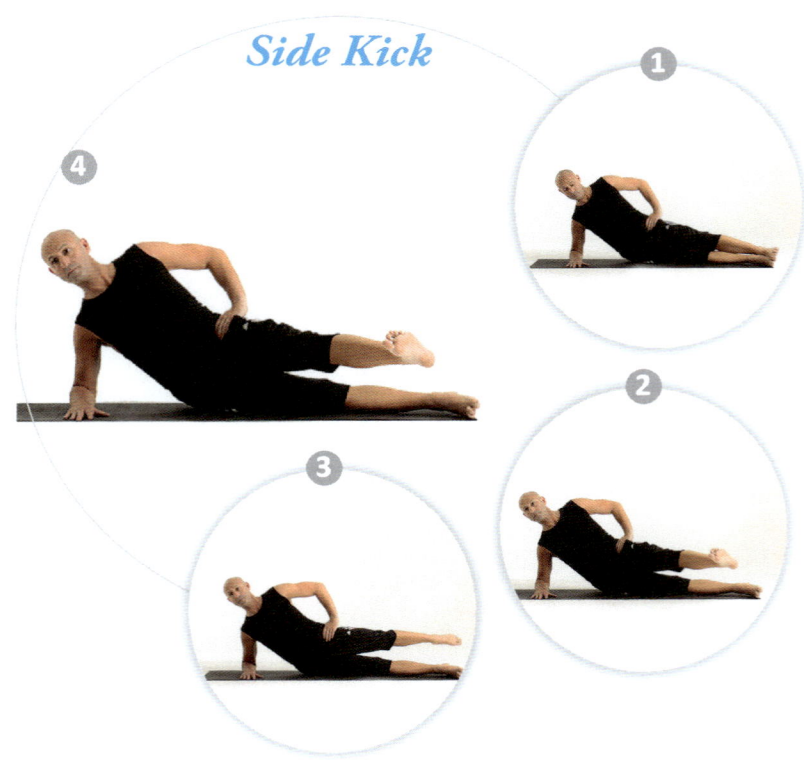

Side Kick

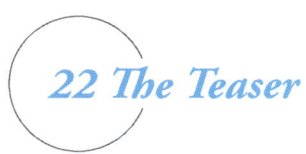

22 The Teaser

Part A — Classical exercises

BACKGROUND

The teaser is a difficult exercise for strength, balance and control. In terms of flexibility, a degree of suppleness in the hamstrings is required. More important, as previously discussed, is to counter balance the work performed by certain muscle groups. In daily life we tend to overuse the flexor muscles, so after this exercise, we will recommend some "companion" stretches.

Major joints and muscles

The hips are in flexion. Try any of the hamstring stretches from **Chapter Two** to facilitate this difficult position. If your school requires a neutral spine during the exercise, the hamstrings will need even greater length than if your instructor allows a flexed trunk and pelvis. In addition, the latissimus dorsi will require length if you wish to hold a neutral position. If they are tight, they will extend the lumbar spine as you flex the shoulders. Perform **stretch 53** for the lats before this exercise.

Counterposes should include a hip flexor stretch and a quadriceps stretch for the legs. Try **stretch 25**.

To relax the spine muscles, which work strongly during the teaser, try rotation and flexion. If you can do the Teaser, chances are your standard is high, so try the more difficult exercises. For rotation try **stretch 38** and for flexion try **stretch 40** part B.

The Teaser

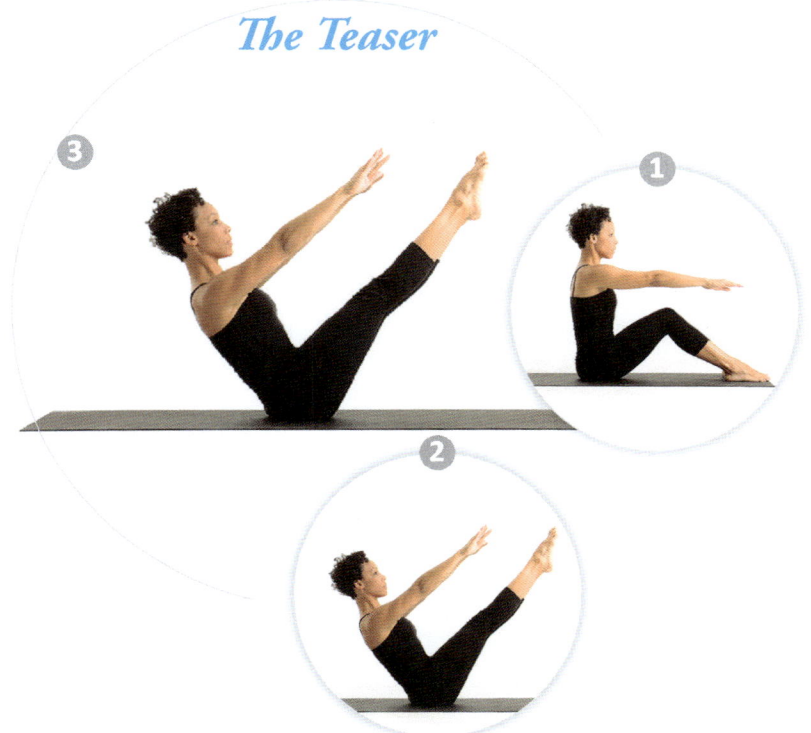

23 Hip Twist with Stretched Arms

**Part A
Classical exercises**

BACKGROUND

This exercise requires various combinations of isometric and isotonic work through the arms, chest, spine, and legs. The hip flexors work strongly to lift and move the legs, the abdominals to stabilise the trunk and the quads to maintain straight legs. Hundreds of muscles are involved in the exercise, but we'll look at the primary ones for stretching and relaxation.

Major joints and muscles

The hips are flexed, so as usual stretch the hamstrings to facilitate this position. Anything from **Chapter Two** will suffice.

The shoulders are retracted, so stretch the anterior deltoid and pectoralis minor to facilitate this. Try **stretch 56 the Lying Bicep**.

Counterpose. Try **stretch 42 the Cobra pose** for a nice counterpose for the muscles of the spine, neck and abdomen.

A **counterpose** for the lats and triceps, which both work hard during the exercise, is **stretch 58**. You could also try the sidebend on the foam roller to stretch out the oblique and QL muscles using **stretch 49**.

Reward the hip flexors and quadriceps with **stretch 23**. Lengthen the adductors, which work hard to keep the legs together, with **stretch 24**.

Hip Twist with Stretched Arms

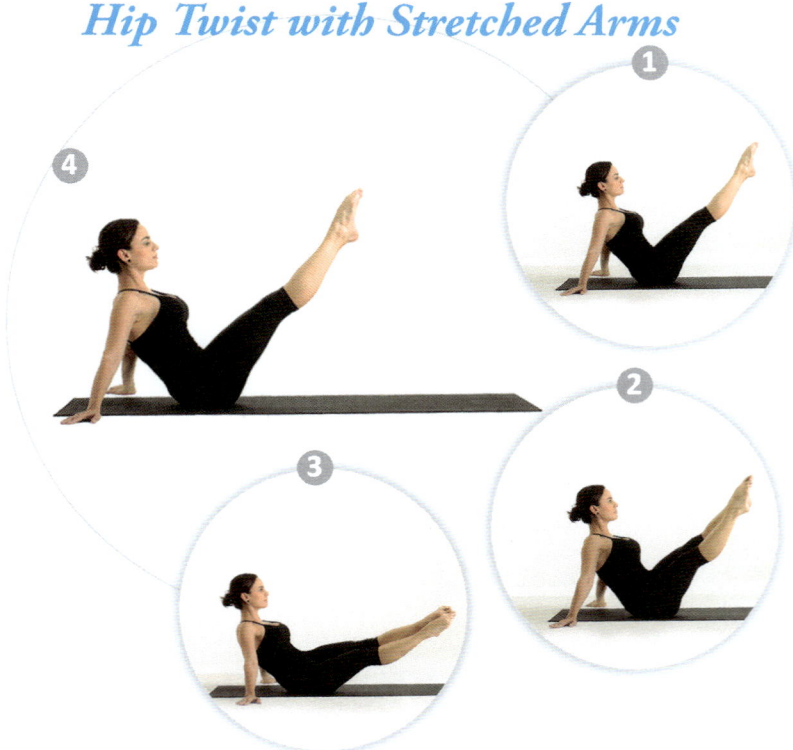

24 Swimming

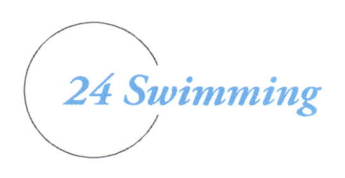

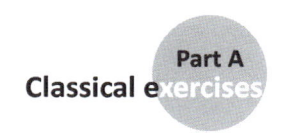

**Part A
Classical exercises**

BACKGROUND

Swimming requires lifting the arms and legs on opposite sides of the body. This requires strength, but tension in the hip flexors and anterior chest wall will make the strength demands far greater. You must stretch the muscles on the anterior side of the body to facilitate lifting the arms and legs and safeguard the lower lumber spine from excessive extension and compression. Both the hip flexors and lats will extend the lumber spine and fascia if they are stiff, causing possible micro trauma and lumbar pain over time.

Major joints and muscles

The hips are in extension. Stretch the hip flexors both before and after this exercise with **stretch 26**. This will also facilitate a stronger gluteus maximus contraction through the process of reciprocal inhibition, described in the introduction to Part B.

The shoulders are technically in "flexion" when you lift the arms. To facilitate this movement, stretch the following muscles groups: the lats with **stretch 53** from Chapter Seven, and the pectoralis major with **stretch 55**.

For a **counterpose** we suggest the very relaxing **box Dangler stretch 38**.

You may also like **stretch 37 the Accelerator** for the mid back.

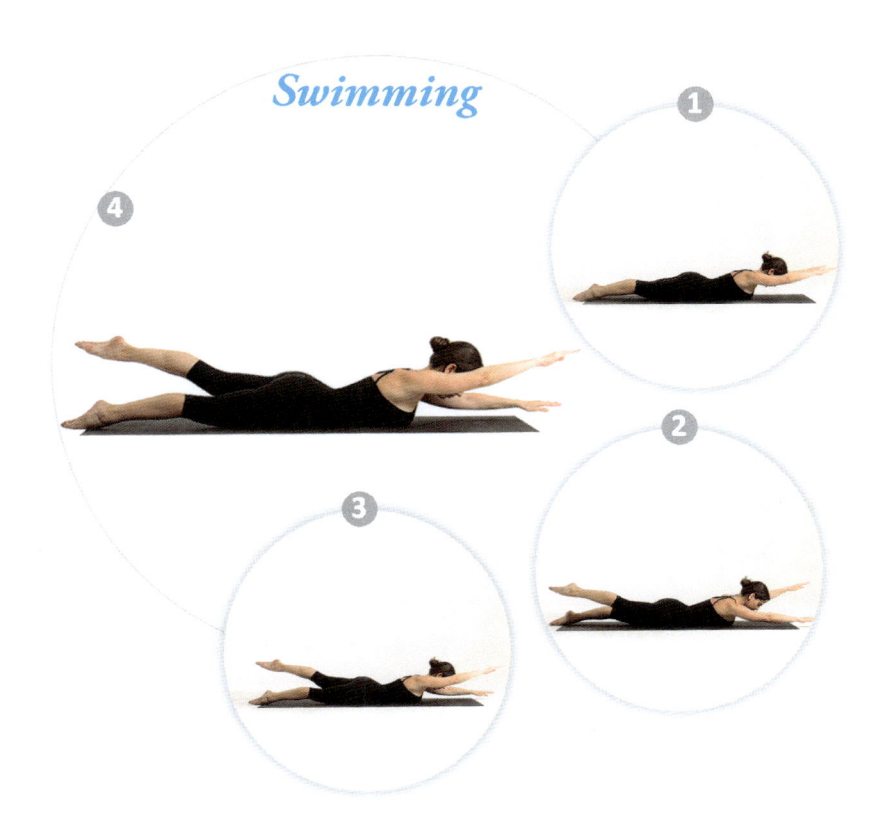

Swimming

25 Leg Pull Front

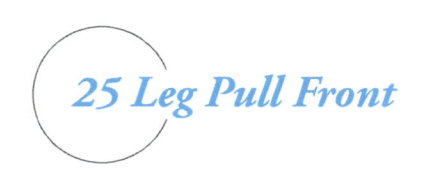

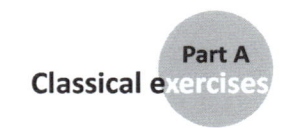

Part A
Classical exercises

BACKGROUND

The Leg Pull Front requires strong shoulder and abdominal stability and gluteal strength. Resistance to the leg lifting is from the hip flexors, and the shoulder girdle works hard to support the trunk. The abdominal muscles also work in this capacity. Try a preparatory stretch for the hip flexors and some counter poses for the shoulders and abdominals.

Major joints and muscles

The hips move into extension. Try any of the hip flexor stretches from **Chapter Three** to facilitate the extension and enable strong firing of the gluteus maximus, the primary hip extensor muscles. Tight hip flexors mean the lumbar spine is forced into extension, causing discomfort and possible strain.

The shoulders work strongly to maintain scapula positioning. Relieve them with a **counterpose** for the middle trapezius and rhomboids. The best stretch for this is the **Pull and Push stretch 48**.

A satisfying counterpose for the shoulders is the internal and external rotator cuff stretches. Find both of them in Chapter Eight, **stretches 60** and **61**.

To relax the pec major, perform **stretch 54**.

A lying backbend to relax the abdominal muscles is the **BOSU Back Bend stretch 41**. If you feel like doing more shoulder work, try the **Cobra stretch 42**.

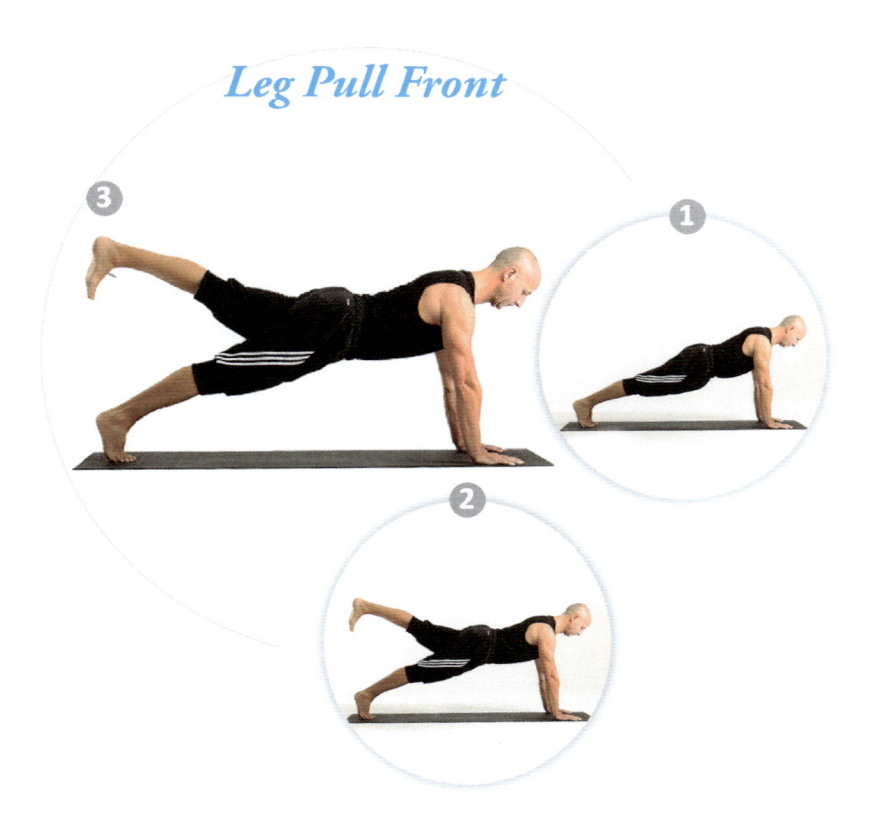

Leg Pull Front

26 Leg Pull

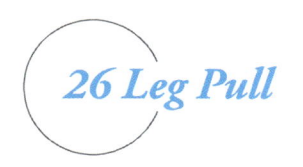

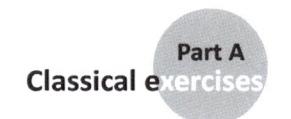

**Part A
Classical exercises**

BACKGROUND

The second stretch in the leg pull series requires significant hamstring and calf length, plus broadness through the front of the chest. The hip flexors also work hard, so we will reward them with a counterpose afterwards.

Major joints and muscles

The hip is in flexion requiring length throughout the hamstrings and calves. Try the **Lying Calf stretch 3** from Chapter One first, followed by **hamstring stretch number 13**.

The shoulders are in extension, requiring suppleness in the anterior chest muscles. Try the **pectoralis major stretch 55** followed by the **pectoralis minor stretch 57**.

For a **counterpose**, reward your hip flexors with the **partner stretch 20** on the foam roller. Reward your spine with the **Accelerator stretch 37** to decompress the lower joints and relax the erector spinae, which work isometrically to hold you in position.

The lats and obliques muscles will also appreciate a counterstretch. Try the **Seated Side Bend 52**.

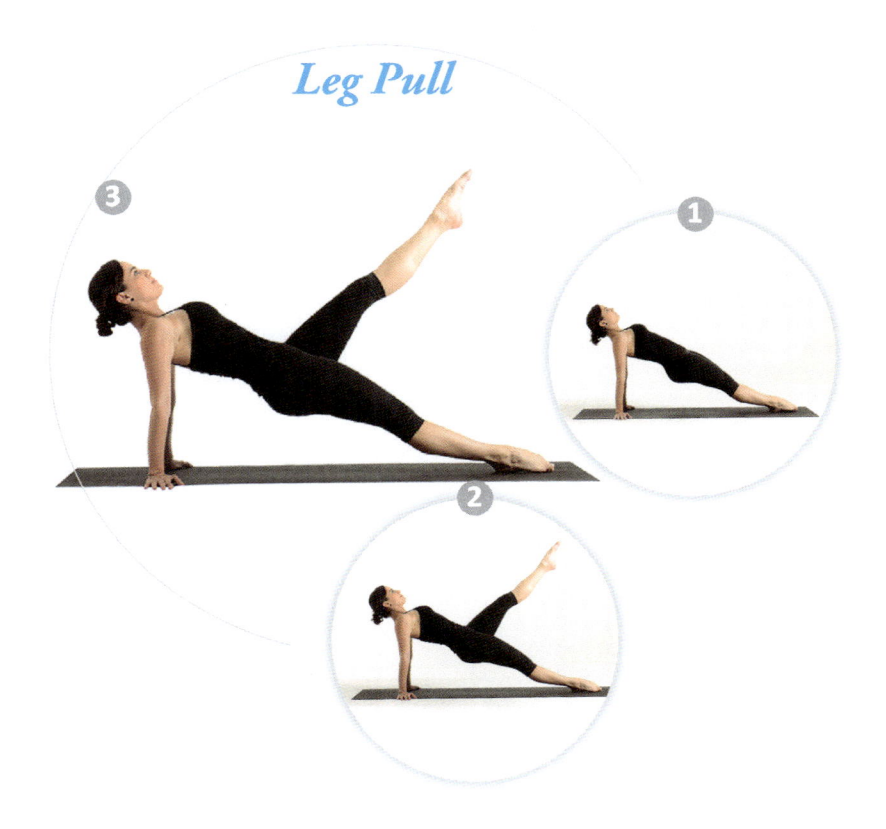

Leg Pull

27 Side Kick Kneeling

**Part A
Classical exercises**

BACKGROUND

This exercise demands greater strength and control than the more simple side kick. That's why Kenyi is demonstrating!

The top leg swings forward and backward demanding flexibility through the hamstrings, gluteus maximus, adductors and hip flexors. A variation includes circumduction of the top leg, requiring greater adductor and abductor flexibility.

Major joints and muscles

The hips are in various stages of flexion, extension, adduction and abduction.

First, stretch the hamstrings with **stretch 15**. Stretch the hip flexors with **stretch 26**. Next, work on the gluteals. **Stretch 20** will cover the glutes, adductors magnus and provide another stretch for the hamstrings and hip flexors.

Finally, work at the adductors with the straight-leg wall **stretch 34**. This targets all the adductors, both short and long.

A **counterpose** for the lateral waist muscles will make relaxing after this difficult exercise easier and prevent soreness the following day. If you're able to do the Side Kick Kneeling, chances are you can do the floor version of the Side Bend too. Look at **stretch 50** and give it a try.

The lateral hip muscles also work strongly during this exercise. Try **stretch 29**, it will relax them all.

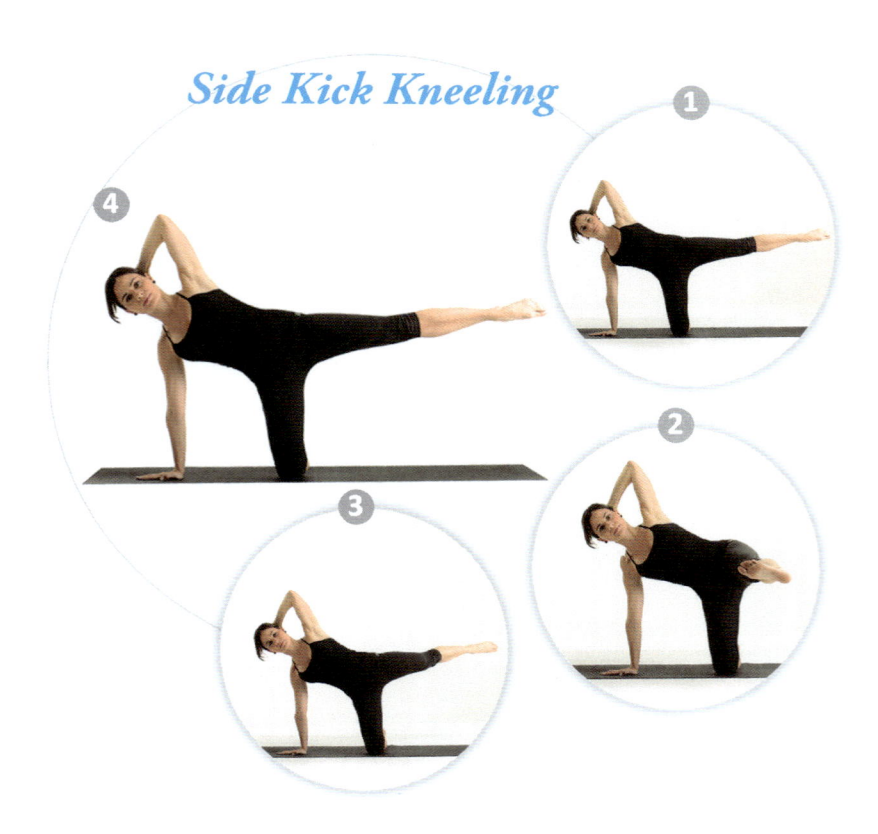

Side Kick Kneeling

28 Side Bend

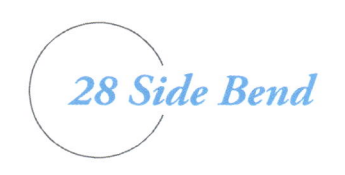

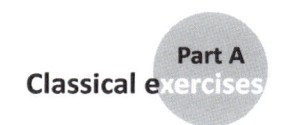

**Part A
Classical exercises**

BACKGROUND
The side bend challenges flexibility through the side of the body – called lateral flexion. It also requires strength to lift you into the correct position. if you have stiffness in your sides, greater strength will be required to overcome this stiffness and achieve a good position. Lengthen the obliques abdominal muscles, the erector spinae, lats and quadratus lumborum to facilitate a more graceful and fluid performance of the exercise. Some thoracic rotation is also required. Try **stretch 46 the Lying Rotation** from Chapter Six as a facilitating stretch.

Major joints and muscles

The spine is lifted into lateral flexion. In preparation, try the **Seated Side Bend stretch 51** from Chapter Six. This is perfect preparation, particularly if you have a partner who can include the lats variation with you. Prolonged practice of these stretches will facilitate far greater success with the Side Bend.

If your lats feel tight, try **Kneeling Lats stretch 53** as an alternative or in addition to the **Seated Side Bend stretch 53**. For thoracic rotation try **stretch 45** as a facilitator.

A **counterpose** for the quadratus lumborum is well advised. Try **stretch 50**. In addition, release the gluteus medius with **stretch 30** or the stronger **version 31**.

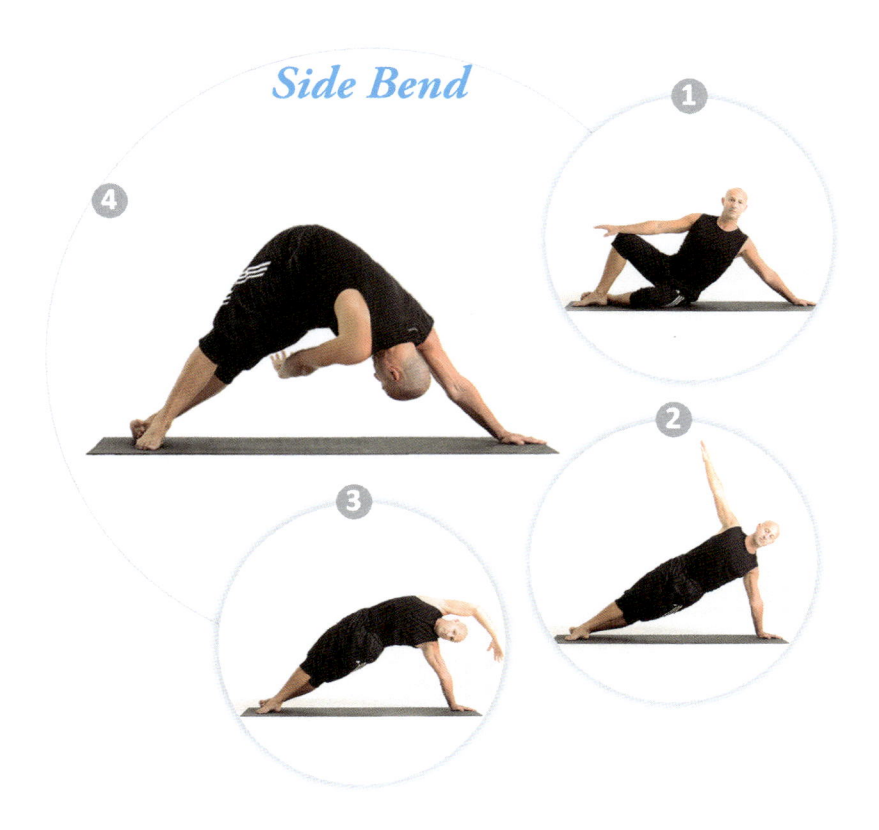

Side Bend

29 The Seal

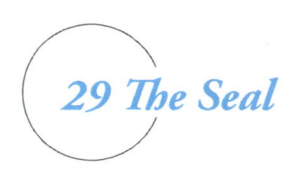

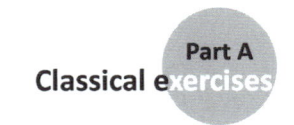

Part A
Classical exercises

BACKGROUND

Predominately the Seal requires balance and control; however, some adductor length is needed throughout and the spine is flexed strongly too. When finished, be sure to add an abdominal and spinal extension stretch to counteract the flexion bias.

Major joints and muscles

The hips are abducted and externally rotated. In particular, the short hip adductors need length because the knees are bent, reducing the tension in the long/two joint adductors like gracilis and the medial hamstrings. **Stretch 32 the Frog** is the perfect preparation as it targets these muscles precisely.

The spine is flexed. Try **stretch 40** to prepare it and the gluteus maximus.

A lovely **counterpose** for the Seal is the **Cobra stretch 42**. It requires strength but moves the lower back, hips, chest, abdominals and neck in the opposite direction to the Seal.

In addition, the external hip rotator muscles work hard to hold the leg position. Reward them with the **Criss Cross stretch 28**.

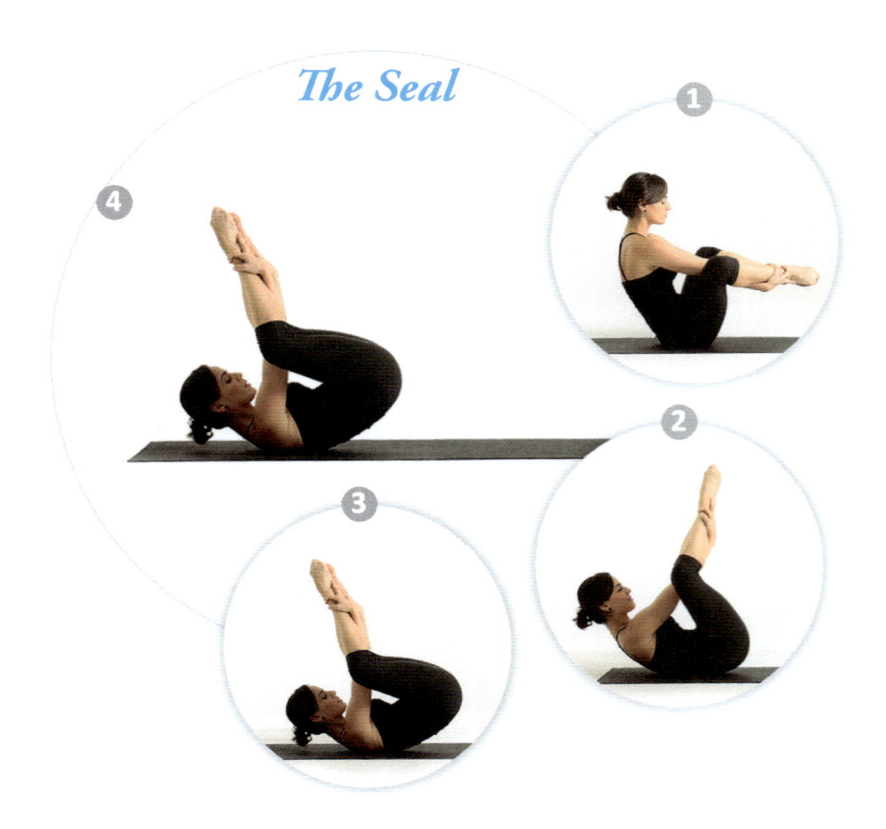

The Seal

30 Rocking

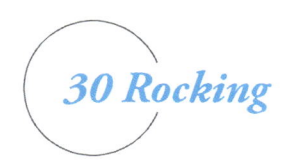

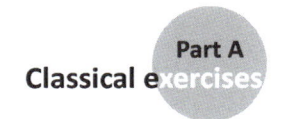

**Part A
Classical exercises**

BACKGROUND

Rocking, as demonstrated below, requires extension flexibility throughout the spine, in the quadriceps, and also in the chest and shoulders. The spine is strongly extended and this position may not be achievable for everyone. Talk to your teacher if you experience pain.

Major joints and muscles

The knees are strongly flexed. To facilitate this, stretch the quadriceps using the floor version of **stretch 25**. This stretches all the quads plus the rectus femoris, which crosses both the knee and hip joint.

Taking hold of your feet requires considerable flexibility in the front of the shoulders, particularly if your arms are not long. If reaching your feet is difficult, your lower back will be forced into further extension.

Try **stretch 57**, which replicates the arm movement of Rocking almost exactly – in particular the variation in photo D.

As a **counterpose,** anything that produces spinal flexion will be worthwhile. **The Dangler stretch 38** is lovely and will decompress the lumber disks, while the **Accelerator stretch 37** will draw apart the shoulder blades. If you have time, do both.

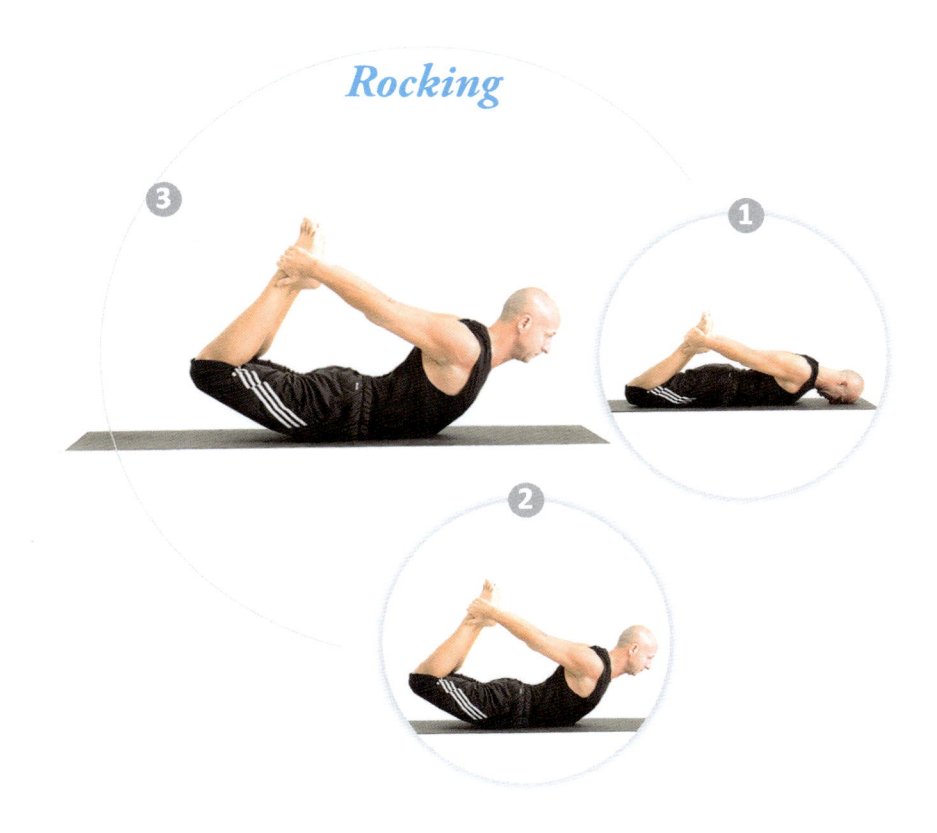

Rocking

31 Control Balance

Part A
Classical exercises

BACKGROUND

Control Balance demands strong neck flexion, spinal flexion and good range of movement through the hamstrings and hip flexors. To raise one leg to vertical, the hip flexors require good length as the pelvis is in posterior tilt. To achieve the pose in the second photograph, the arms and shoulders also require good extension ability.

Major joints and muscles

The hips are both flexed and extended. Attempting this exercise means you are already an advanced student, so go ahead and try the front split in **stretch 72** in preparation. This will stretch both hamstrings and hip flexors strongly. If you are able to do a front split or close to, you have more than adequate flexibility for control balance.

The spine is also strongly flexed. Try the **Foam Roller Hamstring stretch 12** and see if it is comfortable. If so, proceed cautiously to the Control Balance, which is more difficult due to the weight of your trunk bearing down on your neck.

Counterposes would be the **Box Wheel stretch 43** or the **Floor Wheel 44**; another advanced movement, but you are ready!

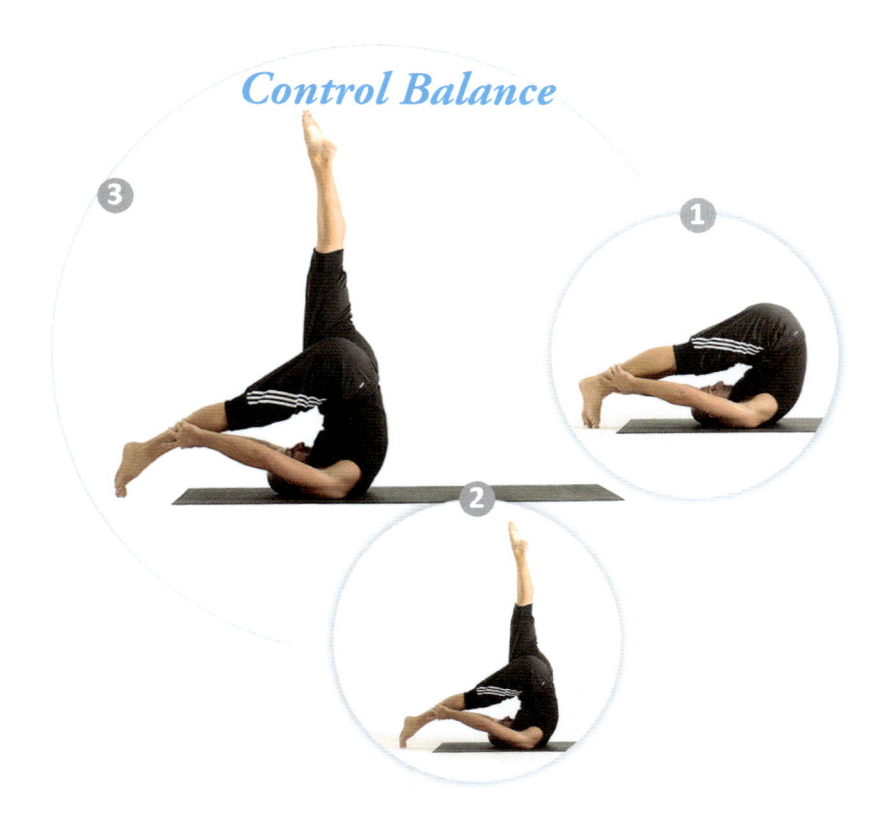

Control Balance

32 Push Up

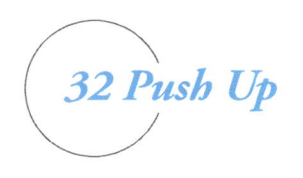

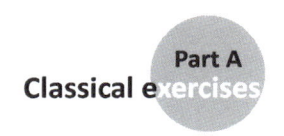

Part A
Classical exercises

BACKGROUND

This unusual combination of movements requires strength and flexibility. The flexibility demands stem mostly from the pose in the second photograph, in which you are required to flex at the hips and touch the floor or mat. Calf, hamstring, gluteus max and adductor longus are stretched here, along with the lumber spine.

Major joints and muscles

The hips are in strong flexion, as are the shoulders. A strong facilitative stretch would be **number 4 the One Leg Dog pose**, which replicates the demands of the Push Up closely. The various positions in the Dog Pose focus on calves, hamstrings, glutes and adductors. It also requires considerable strength in the shoulders, helpful in preparation for the Push Up. Try **stretch 4** in its entirety.

Counterposes for the Push Up should include the **triceps stretch 58** and **pectoralis major stretch 55**.

Both of these muscles work strongly during the exercise. A relaxing backbend would also be lovely. The **Cobra stretch 42** or **BOSU Back Bend 41** from the extension series in **Chapter Six** would be well received by your spine. The hip flexors will also need to relax after stabilising the anterior pelvis. Try **stretch 20**. If you don't have a partner, let one leg hang over the roller and relax.

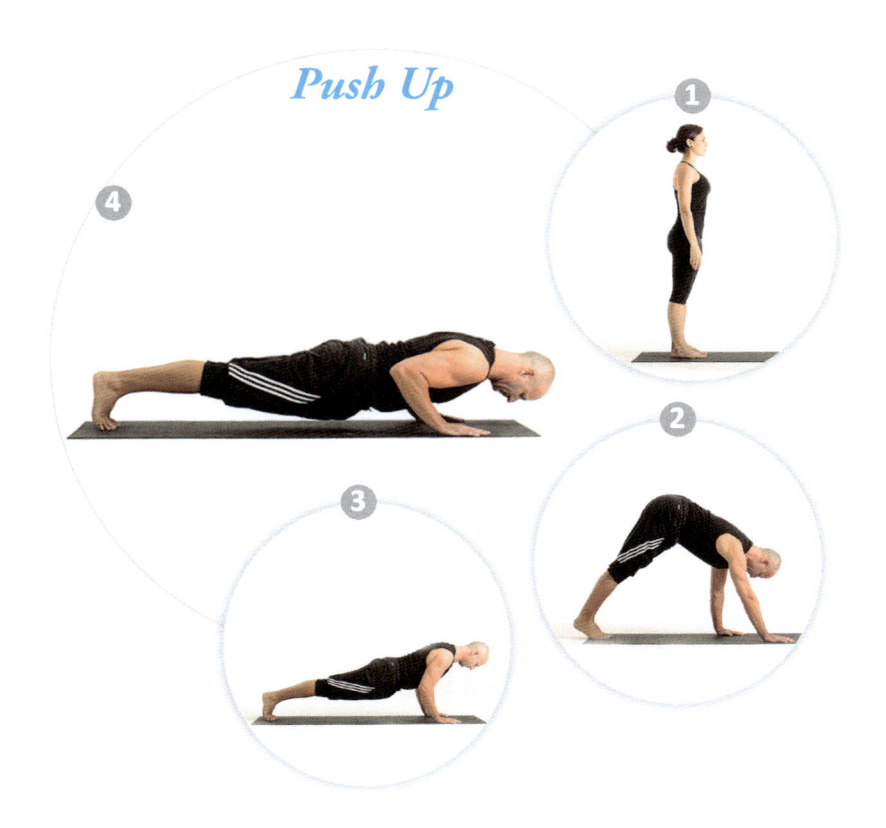

Push Up

Part B
Innovations Stretches

Introduction – Part B

STANDARDS AND VERSIONS

The stretches in part B are not grouped into sections with various standards for two reasons. First, each stretch in itself has degrees of difficulty. You can start with the easiest version and as progress is made increase the degree of difficulty with adjustments in body position. If you don't feel much of a stretch, check that your form is correct. If it is, perhaps you are exceedingly flexible in this particular region. The second reason is that after stretching people for many years, it is our belief that people cannot be generalised into categories. People, and their bodies, are complicated. There are numerous studies that confirm flexibility is not a general characteristic, nor is it uniform throughout the body. In fact, research supports the opposite view: that flexibility is specific to a particular joint. For example, good flexibility in the hip does not ensure adequate flexibility in the shoulder or even in the other hip. (See Alter, *Science of Flexibility* p.3).

In the introduction to part A I quoted Sartre, and it is worth repeating. "We are the authors of ourselves. Through our actions, and our failures to act, we ultimately design ourselves". In the context of stretching, this means that certain repetitive behaviors will have affected our bodies: some behaviors may have caused tightness and restriction, others may have caused freedom and flexibility. So while you may categorise yourself as stiff, this stiffness as a result of certain behaviors is likely confined to particular regions. Similarly, while you may think of yourself as flexible, there will be exceptions. The many ballet dancers that attend my studio provide an example. Although they are generally very flexible, ballet dancers like all of us expose their bodies to repetitive patterns of use or 'stress'. The requirement of turnout (external rotation of the femurs), so critical to classical dance, means that almost every dancer we see has very tight, very strong external rotator muscles. As a consequence, within their mostly lithe and graceful musculature there exist regions of tightness, stiffness and movement limitation.

Although we can predict some outcomes that may follow repeated exposure to particular stresses and behaviours (the governing principle of all physical training from rehabilitation to elite sports training is the SAID principle: 'specific adaptation to imposed demand'), the most general rule that can be made about patterns of flexibility is simply that there isn't one. Your task is to explore slowly and attentively the stretches available here, and discover for yourself where your unique body is both tightest and loosest. In essence, you will be discovering how your body has recorded your activities and experiences.

HOW OFTEN SHOULD I STRETCH?

There is simply no definitive answer to this question. Stretching is a subjective experience that requires exploration. We do not wish to become 'certainty peddlers', advocating all manner of strict practices. A useful distinction, however, is to divide your stretching sessions into 'challenging' and 'restorative' categories. Sessions can be one or the other and, given that range of motion can vary considerably from joint to joint, can also be a combination of both.

Challenging stretches will leave you sore, perhaps for several days. Their purpose is to increase your current range of joint motion or level of flexibility. Delayed onset muscle soreness (DOMS) is the common experience of soreness after such activity, and usually peaks around 48 hours after training. It makes little sense to stretch again while in this state. Repeated stretching or training of already tired muscles (or psycho-physiological stress of any kind for that matter) leads to 'overtraining' or burnout, in which the adaptive or recuperative capacity of the body is exceeded. Remember that your body and its adaptive reserves are finite, and that much of our adaptation to training occurs between, and not during, the session. You must allow your body time to heal. 'Challenging' stretching for increased flexibility is best done two or three times per week per muscle group, with adequate rest factored in to your program.

'Restorative stretching', a title used in Yoga, is different – its goal is psychophysiological relaxation, maintenance, and regaining your current level of flexibility if you feel particularly stiff or sore from prior activity. Restorative stretching can be undertaken more often than challenging stretching – perhaps in the days between bouts of challenging stretching, between challenging stretches in a session you've labelled 'challenging', before sporting activity, or after a long sedentary day. Be aware that while recuperative stretching may *look* the same as challenging stretching, to you it *feels* different. You are not pushing so hard. The most important thing is to tune in to your body and ask yourself how you feel on any given day. Are you tired and in need of relaxation, or is today's session going to challenge and improve your current state?

GOOD FORM

There are two types of form: 'ideal' form and 'good' form. To confuse matters, there is a range of correctness that exists around each of these.

Ideal form is copybook: a stretch that is performed to perfection, one that mirrors exactly the instructions that have been given. Ideal form is the end goal of a stretch and is concerned more with aesthetics – how does the stretch look? Ideal form presupposes a high degree of flexibility to begin with and can be confusing to those who are just beginning stretching.

When your form in a stretch becomes ideal and the stretch can be repeated with relative ease, it is likely that you no longer need to perform that particular stretch. At this point it may be prudent to find a more useful way to spend your stretching time. (Remember, stress drives adaptation. No stress, no adaptation.) Of course, you might still perform the stretch if your goal is to maintain your current state of flexibility, or because you love to perform a particular movement, or even because you like to show off!

Good form is an attempt to emulate ideal form, and is necessary to feel the stretch in those muscles that the stretch was designed for. Without good form you will be doing a different stretch entirely – I sometimes call this 'creative' or 'free-style stretching'. In contrast to ideal form, good form is concerned more with technique – are you positioned so that you can feel the appropriate sensations?

The distinction between good and ideal form is important. Too often teachers insist that a stretch is not correct because it doesn't match the ideal position. But so long as it is biomechanically sound, it is not incorrect – it is simply that the person performing the stretch doesn't have the requisite flexibility (or perhaps the bony architecture) to perform it in a perfect manner at that precise moment. It may still be a 'good' performance, however, in that it resembles the ideal position to a recognisable degree and produces the desired sensations.

Good form is the domain in which we spend most of our stretching lives – trying to elicit certain sensations. This is far more important than attempting to recreate a particular shape in space. Eventually, after many years practice, we may be able to emulate exactly a particular shape. This is pleasing too of course, and gives us a sense of achievement.

The 'range of correctness' is the freedom to explore, within the confines of good form, shifting sensations. Our bodies are covered with muscle and fascia running in a multitude of directions. A slight shift in joint angle will have a corresponding shift in sensation, moving the stretch to tighter bands of muscle fibres within a muscle, or to a particular muscle within a muscle group. (The adductor stretches will give evidence of this range of correctness.) This exploration is enormously important to the process and should be encouraged. Exploration can encourage an inner focus and attention, and engagement with the parts of ourselves that we wish to explore the least: the ones that bring us discomfort and pain. The process of opening up to these regions can be therapeutic, creating awareness: 'food' for further self-exploration, acceptance when it is appropriate, and at other times increasing our determination and desire for change.

WARMING UP

(Increasing body and tissue temperature)

In the sporting arena, warm up has become a specialty and must fulfill certain requirements. The warm up itself must be specific, replicating the unique joint positions and movement patterns of the activity. The goal is not just general 'warmth' and the lubrication of various joints, but more importantly the re-igniting of specific neural patterning and motor skills for the activity, plus adequate blood flow to structures.

When preparing for stretching, your warm up need not be so regimented. You do not need to mimic the actual stretches themselves; any activity that increases body temperature will suffice. More important is that you do not exhaust yourself before your stretching session begins. You need an *efficient* warm up procedure, something that works rather quickly. Wearing warm clothes that do not allow much of your generated body heat to escape is useful, so attend to that first. In winter, I don a 'sauna suit' – a type of nylon tracksuit that traps heat. I look like a walking garbage bag, but it does the trick. Ballet dancers, too, are known for the plastic pants they wear during bar work to increase heat and movement potential.

Once you are dressed, any activity that uses most of the large muscles of the body (gross movements of the arms, legs and trunk) will heat you up in five to ten minutes. Should you warm up for your warm up? No! A warm up is not designed to increase range of movement permanently. Begin slowly, and as you feel your body temperature increase to a mild sweat, gradually up the tempo. Try walking around the block, doing several sets of squats, or performing ten minutes of dynamic Pilates exercises. (Our DVD, 'Innovations in Pilates', has a full warm up sequence on the reformer.) Once you are warm, you are ready to stretch.

Why do we need to warm up? The most direct benefit in warming up for stretching involves decreasing viscosity, or resistance to fluid flow. It is believed that viscosity in muscular and connective tissue is partially responsible for restricting movement. Heat has an inverse relationship to viscosity; that is, as body heat increases, fluid viscosity decreases. This reduced viscosity in turn reduces the resistance to movement and results in increased flexibility.

It is well known that the speed at which nerve impulses travel increases with rising body temperature (recall how clumsy your fingers can be when they are cold). This is probably why most world records are broken in hot environments. When stretching, this translates to more physical control – you are able to feel and manipulate your movements with greater refinement. This is undoubtedly a safer state in which to stretch.

Finally, we should look at more passive forms of warming up. Examples include hot baths, infrared light, massage and various saunas. Passive forms of raising body temperature are more successful than active forms in decreasing muscular tension (improving muscle relaxation). If your goal is to perform a restorative stretching session, combining a passive and relaxing warm up will bring the most positive results. Your nervous system will be 'toned down' and you will achieve greater levels of relaxation. If you have difficulty sleeping, this practice performed before bed may make a tremendous difference.

TYPES OF STRETCHING – REFLEXES

Essentially, stretching involves elongating a group of muscles and fascia by increasing or decreasing the angle around a particular joint or joints. Flexibility is defined as the range of motion available in a joint or group of joints.

When joint movement is performed quickly and continuously at various speeds it is called 'dynamic' or 'ballistic' stretching. When performed slowly it is known as 'static' stretching. An example of stretching statically is bending slowly towards your toes and holding at the point of tension for various periods of time. Performed dynamically, we would bend over and bounce towards our toes for ten or twenty repetitions.

Over the past 20 or 30 years, a great deal of literature has emerged about the merits of different stretching practices and the advantages and disadvantages of each. (See Christopher Norris *The Complete Guide to Stretching* [2004], Aaron Mattes *Active Isolated Stretching* [2000], Michael Alter *Science of Flexibility* [2004], Leon Chaitow *Soft Tissue Manipulation* [1987] and Ayal Lederman *Functional Stretching* [2014] for in-depth discussions on the subject.) As to which method is better, our answer is, as usual, 'it depends'. Different methods of stretching are recommended for different outcomes and the range of considerations is great. How old are you? What is your exercise and health history? Are you stretching before an athletic event, after, or is your desire for flexibility completely unrelated to athletic pursuits? Are you injured? What type of injury? How long have you had the injury? Do you need to learn to relax? Do you want to learn to arouse your body? The adaptations that we make to specific stimuli are highly particular (this is called the 'specificity' principle in sports training) and will affect the type of stretching that we ought to practice. For example, when choosing stretching exercise to improve sports performance we need to match the range of motion, the specific joint angles at which flexibility is required, and the muscles stretched to the actions in the desired sport for it to have maximum benefit. A consequence of such considerations is that until we know the outcome we are seeking, we cannot meaningfully favour one method over another.

For our purposes, to increase the range of movement in our muscles and joints in a safe and efficient manner, static stretching is the most productive method. A study by Wallin in 1985 (Wallin, 'Improvement of Muscle flexibility, a comparison of two techniques', *American Journal of Sports Medicine,* 13.263-268) reported significantly better improvement is the flexibility of the plantar flexors and hip adductors and extensors for those who trained using contract-relax static stretching (up to 25%) compared to ballistic stretching (up to 7%). Why? Because of our primitive muscle reflexes. Reflexes are simple and unconscious motor responses to sensory stimuli carried out at the spinal level, and they bypass higher centres of consciousness. Reflexes are choiceless – they occur in an instant, without conscious effort, and we become aware of them after the event. Several of our body's reflexes are important to the stretching process. Reflexes can both impede and accelerate our progress.

The 'myotatic stretch reflex' occurs when we stretch too quickly (the knee jerk reaction is an example). When the patella tendon is tapped just below the knee cap, the impact stretches the quadriceps muscles on the front of the thigh. The result is a reflexive and protective contraction of the quadriceps that causes the foot to fly up. This reflex is found throughout the body, and its effect on stretching is profound; if you stretch too fast, your muscles will contract. Any dynamic movement activates the myotatic stretch reflex, firing stretch receptors located in muscles, stimulating motor units to shorten muscles, and thereby limiting our ability to stretch. In fact, even thinking about moving results in neuronal activity, stimulating the motor neurons enough to activate at least a few motor units.

Because of this reflex we need to stretch statically, learning to coax and cajole our bodies into giving way. The type of stretching that suits our goals can be likened to the act of going to sleep: it cannot be forced upon us. When we go to bed, we habitually create the conditions that are conducive to sleep – we minimise sensory stimulation, we minimise movement, we slow down our rate of breathing and then we let go. Approaching stretching with this attitude – that is, stretching slowly and without force – will prove far more successful for increasing range of motion than forcing the issue; for instance, as if you were training in a gym. This distinction is an important one: stretching for increased range of motion requires a fundamentally different *attitude* than other forms of exercise training. It requires patience, relaxation and the directing of your attention inward to what is happening inside you. (In *Job's Body*, Juhan describes the myotatic stretch reflex: 'one of the fundamental jobs of the muscle's sensory system is to resist sudden change in muscle length ... this resistance is enforced by an automatic reflex that cannot be bullied ... only slow, patient unthreatening pressure and stretches can avoid triggering more contractile responses.')

In contrast to the myotatic stretch reflex, another of our stretch reflexes, known variously as the 'clasp knife reflex', 'post-isometric relaxation' or 'autogenic inhibition', can be used to our advantage. It causes the targeted muscles to relax rather than contract. The stimulus for the activation of this reflex is not a dynamic movement, but contractile tension in a muscle(s). To activate this reflex, we simply contract a muscle while we are holding it statically in a stretched position. Golgi tendon organs, located near musculotendinous junctions, will react when we do this, reflexively causing the muscle to relax. This feedback loop, in which the contraction of a muscle shuts down its own activity, acts like a thermostat shutting off the heat when the temperature rises. It has a protective function, preventing a muscle from contracting so hard that it pulls its attachment off the bone. (Dis-inhibition is the name given to the suppression of this reflex, and this occurs during the first few months of strength training. During this time, heavier resistances can be lifted even though muscles have not really grown. One's nervous system is 'allowing' the greater recruitment of motor units.)

The clasp knife reflex was discovered by neurophysiologist Herman Kabat and his associate Henry Kaiser and physical therapist Dorothy Voss. In the 1950s they established nine techniques for rehabilitating the muscles of paralysed patients. They called their work 'proprioceptive neuromuscular facilitation' (PNF). Contract/relax (C/R) is the name given to the activation of the clasp knife reflex in their system. (C/R is also known as 'muscle energy technique' in the fields of osteopathic and chiropractic medicine. See Leon Chaitow *Soft Tissue Manipulation*.)

CONTRAX – RELAX

In practice, the contract/relax (C/R) technique is simple. First, the stretcher lengthens the muscle to be stretched. The muscle is taken slowly (so as not to activate the myotatic stretch reflex described above) to the **point of tension (POT)**. The position is held for approximately five deep breaths (25 to 30 seconds) while the stretcher is encouraged to settle and relax (remembering that even thinking about moving will fire some motor neurons).

Second, the stretchee isometrically contracts the muscles being stretched for five seconds. (An isometric contraction is when a group of muscles is activated or contracted and the effort matched by an opposing force so that no actual movement occurs. The opposing force is often a partner.) The degree of force that the stretcher uses can vary. Chaitow recommends no more than 25% to 30% of one's maximum strength, whereas Goodridge ('Muscle energy technique: Definition, explanation, methods of procedure', *Journal of American Osteopathic Association*, [1981]) recommends using larger force for larger muscles and very little force for weaker, shorter and smaller muscles. In our experience, up to around 50% of one's maximum force yields the best results, with force beyond this not making any significant difference to the outcome. However, you need to start with minimum force and build to the 50% force over the five-second period.

Third, after the contraction the stretchee relaxes, takes a deep breath, and on exhalation moves the limb slowly into a deeper, stronger position. This new position is then held for a minimum of ten deep breaths. The degree of restretch can vary, and it is our experience that the more you perform this work, the further the restretch will be. Your body 'learns' to relax. At first, be satisfied with increases of 1 to 5 millimetres. Over time the restretch, measured in angular or linear units, may increase. According to McAtee (*Facilitated Stretching* [2007], p.16), exhaling as you restretch is important – your body is more relaxed and muscles have slightly less tone during this moment. Our practice supports this assertion.

To perform one iteration of the C/R method the hamstring is taken into a position of mild discomfort and then the 5–5–15 timing sequence begins. The initial position is demonstrated below. The position is held for a minimum of five deep breaths.

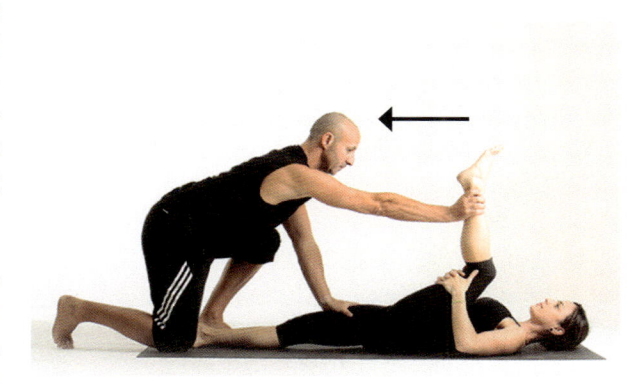

A contraction is performed at 30–50% of one's maximum capacity for five seconds. The contraction direction is demonstrated by the black arrow above.

After the contraction, the stretchee relaxes, takes a deep breath in, and on a breath out restretches to a new position for fifteen deep breaths. (Note that the new position is not necessarily more uncomfortable. In fact, the 'rate of perceived exertion' (RPE) should be much the same as before the restretch.) The restretch is demonstrated in the photo on the following page.

This explains one iteration of the C/R procedure. You can try up to three iterations for greater effect.

RECIPROCAL INHIBITION

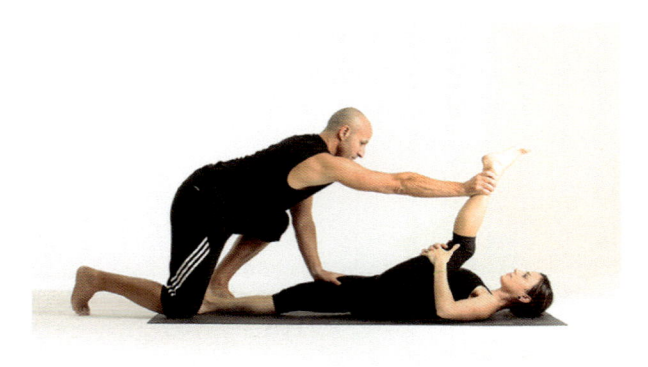

Reciprocal inhibition or innervation (RI) was discovered by Sir Charles Sherrington in 1947 in the development of a model for how the neuromuscular system works. RI is another involuntary reflex that can affect our stretching practice. When a muscle contracts, for example the *biceps* of the arm, RI occurs to inhibit its opposing muscle the *triceps* from contracting also, because this would prevent any movement whatsoever. The value of this reflex is twofold: it can be useful both prior to and just after stretching any muscle group. When restretching after a contraction, we can use the *opposing* muscle group whenever possible to produce the movement. For example, when stretching the hamstrings we use the quadriceps and hip flexors to further increase the stretch after a contraction. In doing so we use RI to reduce the nerve impulses to the muscles we are stretching and therefore reduce their resistance to elongation.

Just prior to stretching we can use RI to relax the targeted muscles. For example, a contraction of the quadriceps just prior to stretching the hamstrings may reflexively relax the hamstrings. This is common practice in osteopathic medicine.

RI has implications for Clinical Pilates, and also any form of corrective exercise. Good posture and alignment is dependent on the balance of muscular forces around our joints. For example, rounded shoulders and a poking chin (known as upper crossed syndrome) are the result of an imbalance of forces around the shoulder girdle. Most commonly, the upper part of trapezius, levator scapulae, pectoral and biceps muscles are tight and short, while the deep neck flexors and lower scapular stabilisers are inhibited and weak. In correcting such an imbalance we cannot simply strengthen the weak muscles. Why? Because of the RI reflex. In this instance, the tight muscles of the chest are inhibiting the muscles on the other side of the joints, reducing their tone (by reducing the number of nerve impulses reaching the muscles) and preventing their ability to become stronger. This effect, called 'pseudoparesis', is a dominant feature of muscle imbalance around joints and necessitates the stretching of tight muscles before any type of corrective strength procedure can be effective. Dr Craig Leibenson in the influential *Rehabilitation of the Spine* makes the point: "In rehab it is important to identify and correct overactive and short musculature prior to attempting a muscle strengthening regimen ... the effectiveness of any rehab program is enhanced if hypertonic muscles are relaxed, and stretched prior to initiating a strengthening program."

The body's reflexes are complex and often seem overwhelming. Indeed, when discussed in abstraction their processes can be difficult to grasp. In practice, however, they can be used in a simple fashion to enhance our stretching pursuits. Stay with us and we will make both sense of them, and use of them, before long.

A fourth type of body reflex is worthy of a brief mention too. The 'automatic flexion' reflexes are engaged when we experience pain and fear. The reflexive reaction to hearing a loud bang or touching something hot is almost without exception to withdraw, flex and even move towards the fetal position! I mention this reflex because I am sure it has a role in our patterns of muscle stiffness. If we are repeatedly exposed to anxiety and tension, either of a physiological or psychological nature, or if we are perhaps a little fearful or moderately stressed all of the time, it is logical that the muscles involved in the flexion reflex will become adaptively shortened. Many clients show this: shoulders up around their ears, chests sunken, hip flexors shortened after a day of bracing themselves against an inhospitable world. Our work will be of tremendous benefit to them.

BREATHING DURING STRETCHING

In the breathtaking (if you'll pardon the pun) *Anatomy of Hatha Yoga* [2002], Coulter describes four different kinds of breathing – paradoxical, thoracic, abdominal and diaphragmatic – and the relationship of each to the practice of stretching or Hatha Yoga. It is beyond the scope of this book to investigate this subject in great detail, but the way in which posture (or position) affects breathing and how breathing affects posture is fascinating and complex.

During your practice there will be positions in which your breathing feels restricted and others in which you are able to breathe more fully. Do not be alarmed, this is normal; breathing depends on the position of the body and which parts of it are fixed or relaxed, and the effect that this has on the diaphragm. Leslie Kaminoff in his book *Anatomy for Yoga* elaborates on this process by describing breathing as "shape change in the body's cavities". This brilliantly simple explanation can be observed while you stretch. Parts of the two cavities most affected by breathing, your rib cage and your abdomen, will change shape according to their capacity to do so. Because the diaphragm has multidimensional action, the type of movement, and therefore shape change it produces, depends on which region of its attachment is stable and which is mobile. It can produce belly bulging, rib cage lifting or a combination of the two. In a supine stretch, for example, the top of the dome of the diaphragm is pulled straight down like a piston, with the chest wall acting like a cylinder. The abdominal wall stretches out anteriorly (forward) as the diaphragm descends, and moves backwards (downwards) as the diaphragm relaxes and rises during exhalation.

Side bending provides a different experience, a kind of half belly-bulge with some rib cage expansion. Because the lower half of the abdomen and ribcage are compressed on the side you are bending toward, the downward movement of the dome of the diaphragm is impeded. Because the abdominal organs are liquid and cannot be compressed they act as a fulcrum, causing the diaphragm to cantilever its costal site of attachment on the rib cage outwardly, spreading the base of the ribcage to the front, rear, and sides on the side you are stretching.

Whether you feel a belly bulge or a rib cage expansion or both, breathe as deeply as possible in all of the stretches. Concentrate on your breathing as well as the stretch; this will intensify your experience of the stretch by encouraging an inner focus: an "inhabiting" of your body.

Initially, particularly if you are new to stretching, your focus should be on smooth, even, slow and quiet deep breathing. Breathing in such a manner is relaxing, and relaxation is a psycho-physiological experience. The more relaxed you can become, the less resistant your muscles will be to being stretched. Deep breathing has profound healing effects too. Herb Benson's book *The Relaxation Response* was a groundbreaking work on the subject, and details many of the positive neurophysiological responses to breathing and relaxing.

Make sure that your breathing does not become shallow and constricted. Shallow breathing is with the upper chest – the normal rise and fall of the abdomen does not take place and the lower part of the sternum and the lower ribs don't move. In shallow breathing, the only real sign of inspiration is in the rise and fall of the clavicles (collar bones). "Habitual upper chest breathing", says Coulter, "not only reflects physical and mental problems, it creates them". Indeed, repeated shallow breathing stimulates the "flight or fight" response, raising heart rate and blood pressure, causing muscle tension and leaving you feeling anxious. In addition, constricted breathing is ineffective; it delivers the bulk of the air intake to the upper part of your lungs, the part that is most poorly supplied with blood. And finally, constricted breathing overworks the accessory muscles of respiration, those muscles around your head and neck that we wish to relax. The message seems clear: breathe and relax, breath and relax ...

MUSCLE IMBALANCE

When you start to stretch you will discover, perhaps to your surprise, that your body is not symmetrical. In *Job's Body*, Juhan explains the development of the asymmetry: "It is inevitable that we develop anomalies, because we will never use our bodies symmetrically". Intuitively, we all know the truth of this comment. Even with the best of conscious intentions, it would be nearly impossible to use our bodies symmetrically – imagine shifting your computer mouse to the other hand on alternate days, or reversing the car out of the garage by turning left instead of right in the second half of each week.

Another obstacle to using our bodies symmetrically is that we are creatures of habit, driven to accrue motor patterns and acquire them rapidly. These repetitive, ingrained skills free our consciousness for more complex matters – life, after all, would be exceedingly difficult if we had to literally plan every step. In developing unconscious patterns of movement, however, little thought is given to developing muscles symmetrically or how asymmetrical development will affect our health. So what do we do? In practical terms the answer is straightforward – stretch the tighter muscles more often. A simple rule of thumb is that where you have two of the same muscles in your body (e.g. hamstrings), and you find that one is tighter, stretch it twice as often. In a stretching session, stretch the tighter side first, stretch the looser one next, and then return to the tighter one. In time (perhaps two to three months), the imbalances will be resolved.

Outside your stretching sessions you can begin to combat destructive movement habits by using the greater awareness that you have gained during stretching. Juhan expresses this: 'To throw off the development of the degenerative habits that bow and bind us, we need awareness of the tendencies towards which our muscular habits are leading us, awareness of the local areas of the body that are conditioning those tendencies, and awareness of what it would feel like if our patterns were different'.

Stretching can impart this awareness more quickly and directly than any other means. Stretching, if done with attention, enables you to pause, to actually *feel* what has come about through habitual usage, to explore problem areas and most importantly to experience the relief of release.

HOW LONG SHOULD I HOLD A STRETCH

We must overcome two restrictions to become more flexible. The first is neural, or contractile, the second mechanical. Without the protective mechanisms of the nervous system, the muscle fibres, connective tissue and nerves themselves would tear. The contract/relax (C/R) and other neural techniques described previously help us to work with and around this protective system. Mechanically, the muscle fibres and the surrounding connective tissue and fascia must be lengthened.

We have discussed how the nervous system can be tricked. The C/R technique has an immediate effect, allowing joint range of motion to improve instantly. With repeated practice, the brain's image of what is 'normal length' can be reset. This is the neural adaptation to repeated stretching that we wish to encourage. Much of our resistance to stretch is due to early triggering of nervous system activity and restraint becoming 'normal'. This is because of the limited daily activity of our bodies. When using the nervous system to improve our flexibility, we need to perform at least one iteration of the 5–5–15 sequence described previously. However, as we are hoping to affect more than just our nervous system, I'm advocating more repetitions, up to three.

The nervous system and its limitations has a place of course: it warns us through pain of impending tissue damage. When it is entirely shut down, for example under deep anesthesia, muscles become so loose that joints are easily dislocated. Therefore, the nervous system provides the practical limits to flexibility in day-to-day life, and the muscle and connective tissue provide the outermost limits.

Influencing the mechanical limitations to flexibility requires more work. When muscles become lengthened, the filaments move apart and the sarcomeres (units or blocks of filaments) become longer. Over a period of time, repeated stretching of sarcomeres causes the muscle to adapt by increasing the number of sarcomeres. In effect, the muscle grows in length by the addition of numerous little contractile units. It's like adding another link to a chain. (This biological adaptation to a mechanical stimulus is called 'mechanotransduction'.) The connective tissue gradually follows the lead of the muscle fibers, and the muscle as a whole gets longer. Studies of muscles that have been held in casts in stretched positions confirm the growth of sarcomeres and, unfortunately, muscles that are held in foreshortened states (or are not used anywhere near their full capacity) lose sarcomeres and become shorter.

To effect such biological adaptations you must hold stretches for longer than you would like. The 5–5–15 breath cycle described above is the absolute minimum. After a month or two of stretching, when the nervous system response to stretching has been toned down somewhat, up to three iterations of the C/R procedure is preferred, particularly for large muscle groups. Although the neural system can be tricked, the lengthening and growth of muscle and fascia will not be stimulated without prolonged stretching.

ANATOMY

We hope you enjoy the anatomy photos – a picture truly is worth a thousand words. Keep in mind though that every stretch acts upon many muscles, often too many to display. What we've done is select the major muscles being stretched and displayed those with some exciting graphic design. For those interested in further detail, we have included comprehensive muscle charts that you can refer to. These will enable you to check exactly all of the muscles under stretch during any exercise.

TENSION AND COMPRESSION

Tension and compression refer to the two most important sensations experienced when stretching. The terrific Yoga anatomist Paul Grilley introduced me to these ideas in his work *Anatomy for Yoga*. Tension is the feeling of stretching, the lengthening of muscle and fascia, the (mostly!) delicious sensation that accompanies the correct performance of a stretch. Of course tension can become pain, too, if you do not work with sensitivity and within the parameters we describe shortly. Tension is difficult to describe, and people who are new to stretching and not particularly 'in their bodies', so to speak, will describe all manner of sensation as a stretch because they have not learnt to differentiate between the sensations that arise during stretching. **Tension** is the feeling you experience on waking in the morning, when you arch backwards and prepare to arise. It is often observed in the animal kingdom too. Its technical name is *pandiculation*. Picture a cat or dog as they arch forwards or backwards after napping at various times during the day.

Compression is the opposite sensation. Compression describes the experience of joints, tendons, bones, skin and fat as they lock together to prevent movement. Flex or bend your elbow as far as you can and you will feel the compression between your forearm and bicep. (This is often why bodybuilders become so stiff. It is not so much the weight lifting that causes stiffness, but the muscle bulk that prevents movement and over time creates adaptive shortening.)Straighten your arm as much as you can and you will experience compression in the bones of the elbow joint.

In the next few pages we highlight the possible instances in which compression may be experienced during a stretch. Next to these, we include images of the variations in bone structure that explain why compression may occur in some people and not in others. In our workshops we are able to work with individuals, testing for structural differences and the likelihood of compression, following with recommended alternatives. Because of the myriad variations in structure within and between individuals, we cannot do this in a text. Instead, we will alert you to the possibility of compression by demonstrating visually the joint positions in which it might occur.

In some cases compression can cause inflammation and tissue damage over time. Compression in the shoulder joint is an example whereby repeated overhead arm movements can bring about tendinopathies. In other cases compression is not harmful; in fact the compression of a joint can be momentarily beneficial for various reasons. Compression of body fat around the waist during side bending may prevent further stretching, but is not particularly injurious, and the disks of the spine actually rely on movement and compression for hydration and renewal. What is essential is that you understand that *when compression occurs, you may need to try a different approach.* You can try a different stretch, try to move slowly within the stretch to alleviate the feeling of compression, or recognise that in most instances compression is the end of the range of motion of that joint. No further stretching will induce changes in the shape of your bones. You are done, and what's next for you is acceptance! You also need to know that compression is personal – it is not a sign of weakness or failure, and it will vary with, and within, each individual as the anecdotes below will illustrate. It is possible, of course, to experience both tension and compression. In such instances you and your teacher can decide in which direction you should proceed.

ANECDOTES

In my early years as a Pilates student, I was given an exercise called 'Knockey Knees' on the reformer. To perform it, you lie on the carriage with your feet about hip width apart and knees pressed firmly together. You then move the carriage in and out in a pulsing action, 30 to 50 times. The main purpose of the exercise is to strengthen various parts of the quadriceps muscles. In my case I always felt considerable pain in both the knees and hips. I now realise that the pain in my hips was compression of the femur and the hip joint, or acetabulum. The structure of my hip joint does not permit any real internal rotation of my femurs without considerable compressive force. The sensation at my knees was the meniscus complaining about the stress it was experiencing being under load for prolonged periods. My knees experienced a twisting force that they were not well designed to endure. Twenty years later, I have had meniscal surgery on both knees. Of course, other factors contributed to my meniscal degeneration, but the imposition of biomechanically inappropriate forces on my knees and hips could have been avoided with a little knowledge of compression and tension.

Several years ago Kenyi was visited by an unhappy client who was concerned that, after years of practice, he could not sit in full lotus position while meditating. His master had said it was because he did not focus and his practice was not sufficiently earnest. On testing the ability of his hip joints to turn outward or externally rotate (the key requirement to sit in lotus position), it was obvious to Kenyi that his joints were not designed to do so, no matter how much practice he undertook. The moral of the story is that as teachers and students we need to acknowledge tension and compression so as to maximise the effectiveness of our programs and minimise the potential for harm, both psychological and physical.

Compression – the Shoulder Joint

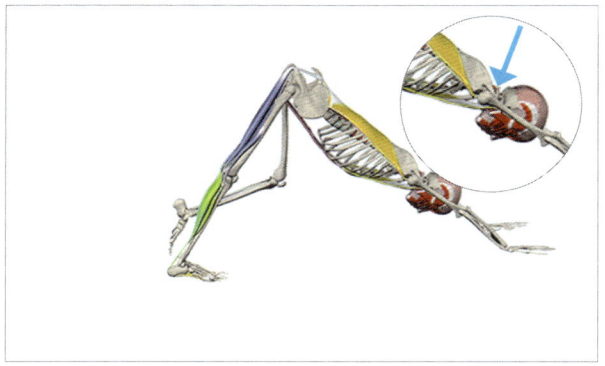

The shoulder joint is the joint in which compression is most often experienced. Any stretch in which the arms are overhead, and in particular load bearing, may bring about feelings of compression deep in the joint. Compression here most often occurs between the acromium and the tissues between either the greater or lesser tubercles. A look at the bone photographs below reveals the remarkable variations in bone shape and size, explaining why some are prone to compression while others are not.

If you experience compression in the shoulder, as a first step try to externally rotate the humerus. This creates space under the acromium process. Second, back out of the stretch a little. Sometimes this will alleviate the problem and force your muscles do do more work, rather than allow the joint collision to support you in the stretch.

Some stretches in which shoulder compression may occur include the One Leg Dog Pose, the Wheel pose, the BOSU Back Bend, the Latissimus Dorsi, the Triceps, Floor and Seated Side Bend, Lying Bicep and Pectoral stretches. Pilates mat exercises with the shoulders in flexion – like the Double Leg Stretch, versions of the Teaser, the Neck Pull and Swimming – have the potential to create compression in the shoulder joint.

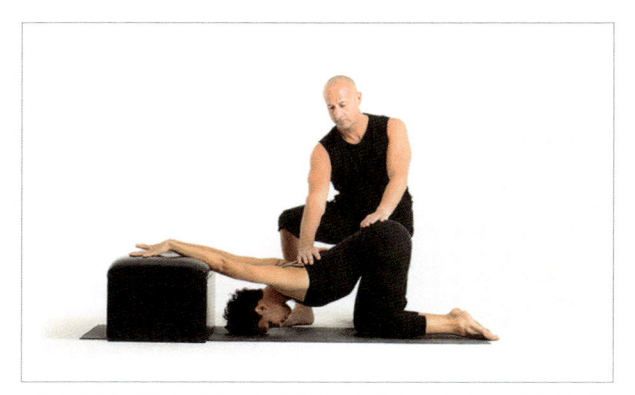

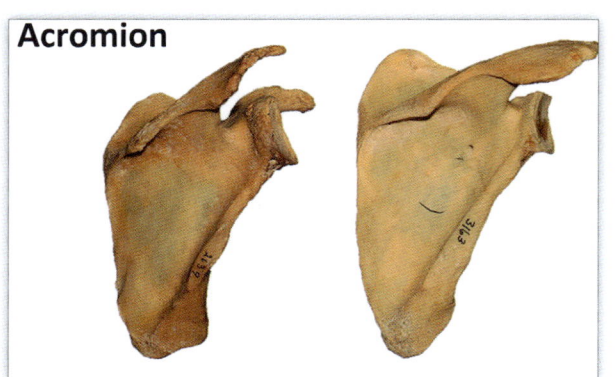

Acromion

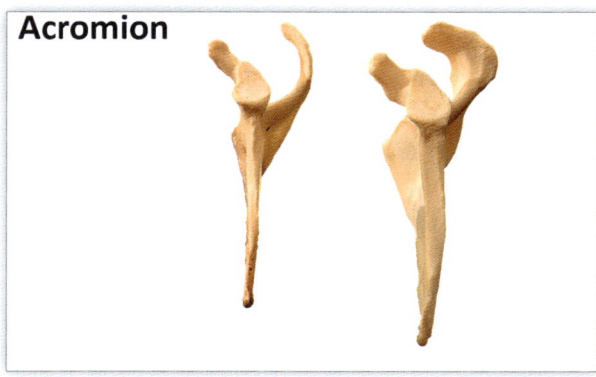

Acromion

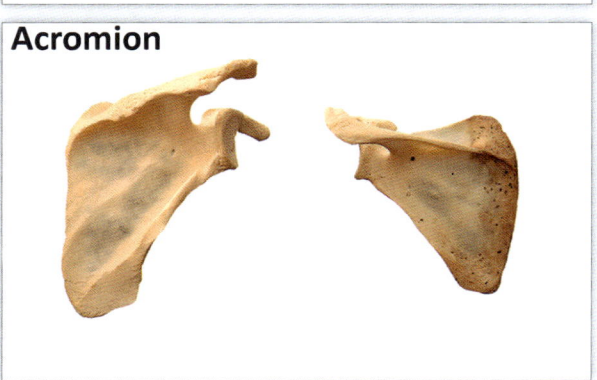

Acromion

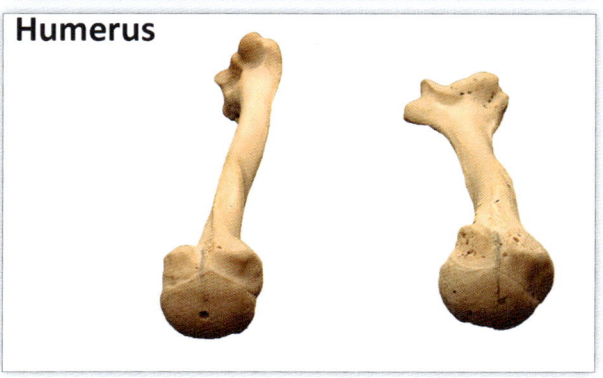

Humerus

Compression – the Hip Joint

The hip joint is another major joint at which compression can occur. Stretches where the leg bones or femurs are abducted or flexed are most likely to create compression sensations. The compression most often occurs in the tissues between the greater trochanter and the hip joint rim called the acetabulum. A look at the bone photographs reveals the diversity of hip and femur shapes. The head and neck of the femur show extraordinary differences, and the angle of the acetabulum too. You can imagine the different movement potentials caused by such variation. Remember that variations can exist within individuals too, so one hip joint can be markedly different to the other.

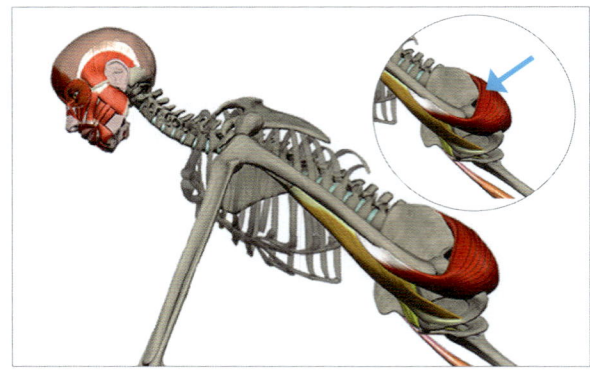

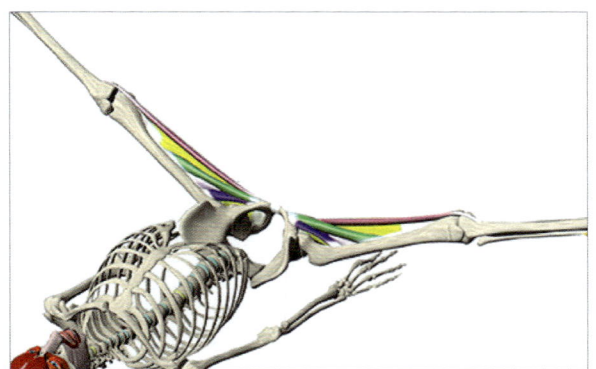

If you experience compression while your hip is in flexion, try abducting it a little. If your compression occurs during abduction, like in the side splits, try externally rotating the femur to create more space in the joint.

Some stretches in which compression may be a factor include all of the adductor stretches in Chapter Four and the lunge poses in Chapter Three. Pilates mat exercises like the Leg Circle, the Seal and the strong hip flexion they require may subject the hip to compression.

Femur

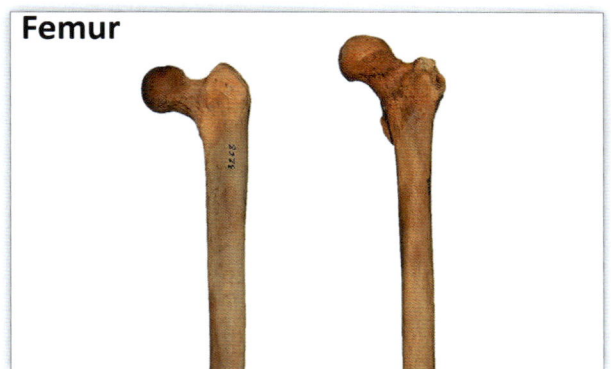

Hip socket

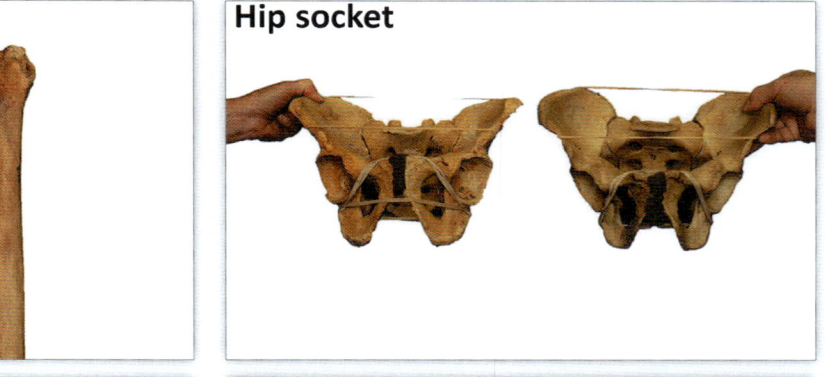

Hip socket

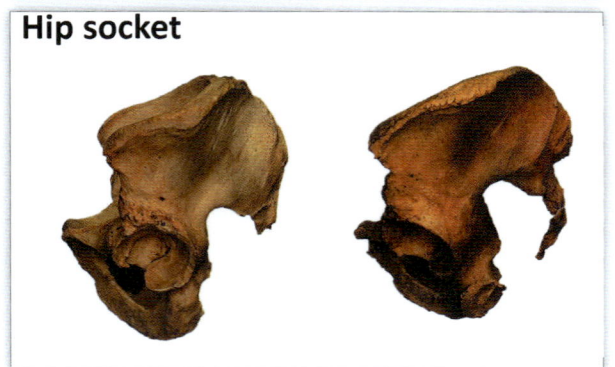

Femur

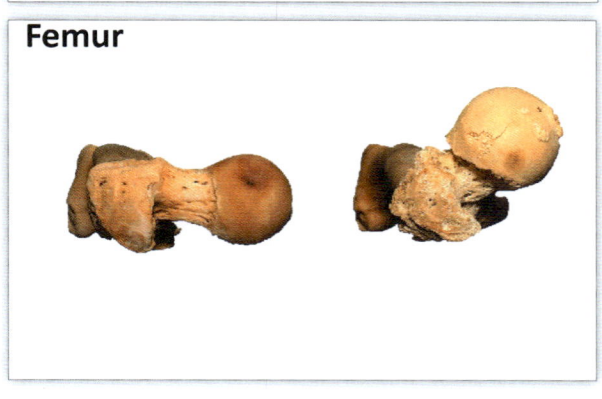

Compression – the Lumbar Spine

The spinous process of the entire spine can be compressed to prevent extension of the spine. In our stretching work it is most often the lumbar spine that is under strong and potentially harmful extension strain. The compression occurs when the spinous processes are jammed together, which can also result in anterior strain on the intervertebral disks.

A look at the bone photograph below reveals that some spines are more capable of extension than others, as the spinous processes have more space between them and permit greater movement. Before attempting a strong back extension exercise like the Wheel Pose pictured at right, it is useful to ascertain the degree of potential mobility of your spine. If compression is a factor, an adaptation may be necessary. In Chapter Six, the Box Wheel is an example in which elevating the feet decreases the degree of lumbar extension. Other exercises, like the Cobra, the BOSU Back Bend and the Latissimus Dorsi stretch may be limited by bony compression.

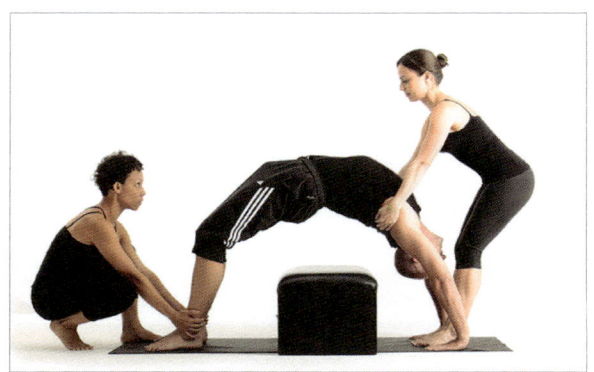

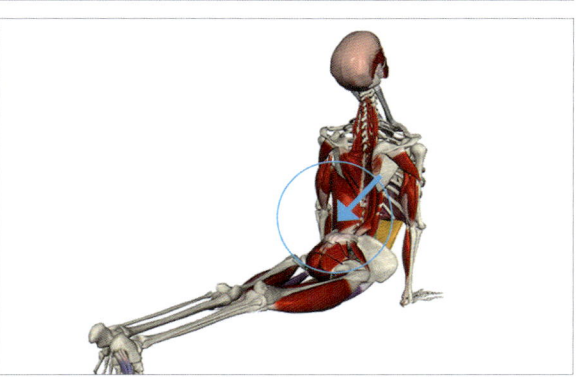

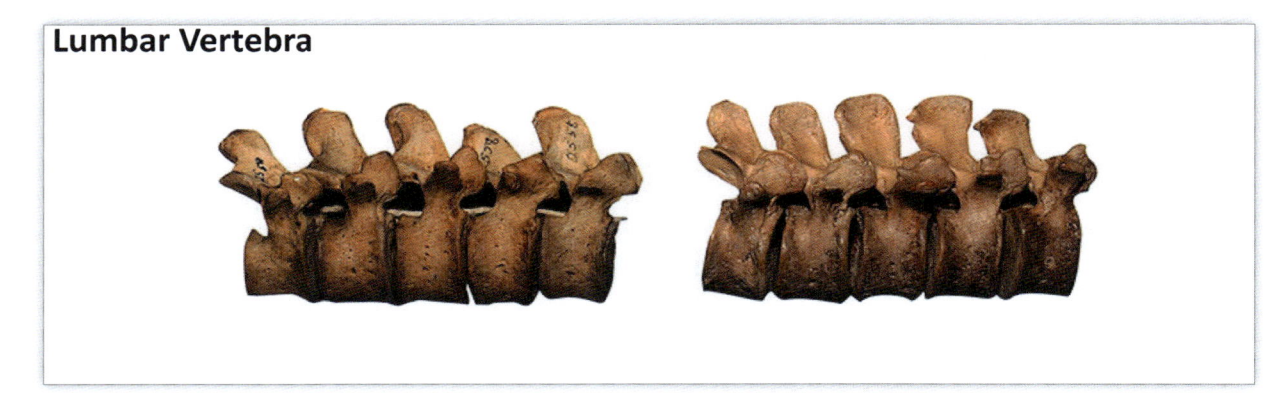

Pilates mat exercises like Rocking, Swan Dive and the Double Leg Kick may also subject the spine to compression.

Lumbar Vertebra

The Calves/Lower Leg/Foot
Chapter 1

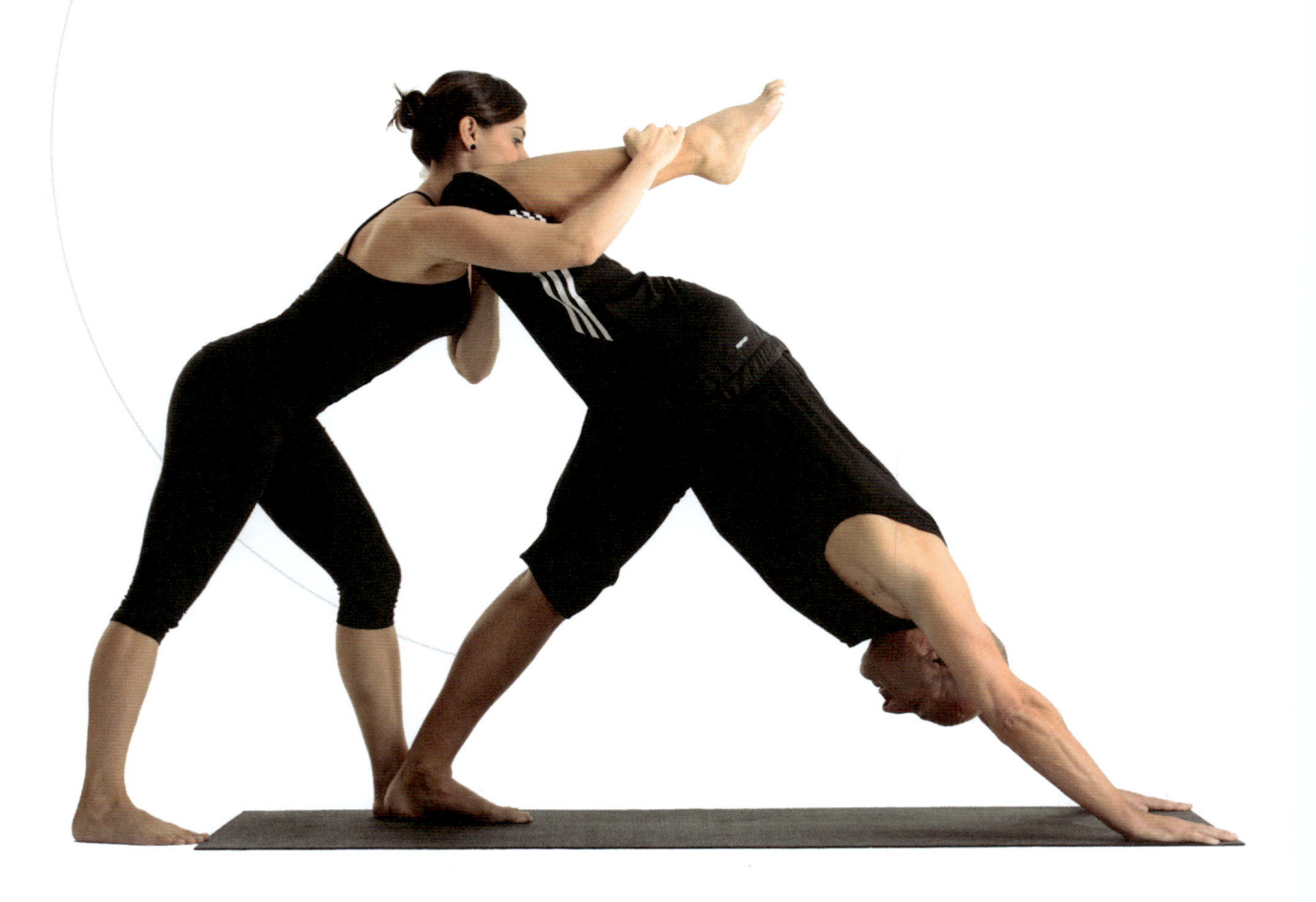

Chapter 1 – Muscle Chart

Foot

Muscle	Toe Flexion	Toe Extentsion	Toe Adduction	Toe Abduction
Flexor digitorum brevis	●			
Flexor hallacus brevis	●			
Flexor digiti minimi brevis	●			
Extensor digitorum brevis		●		
Extensor hallucis brevis		●		
Abductor digiti minimi				●
Abductor hallucis				●
Adductor hallacis			●	
Lumbricales	●	●	●	
Plantar interosseus	●		●	
Dorsal interosseus	●			●

Lower Leg

Muscle	Ankle plantar flexion	Ankle dorsiflexion	Foot eversion	Foot inversion	Toe flexion	Toe extension
Gastrocnemius	●					
Soleus	●					
Tibialis anterior		●		●		
Tibialis posterior	●			●		
Peroneus longus	●		●			
Peroneus brevis	●		●			
Peroneus tertius	●		●			
Flexor digitorum longus	●			●	●	
Flexor hallucis longus	●			●	●	
Extensor digitorum longus		●	●			●
Extensor hallucis longus		●		●		●

Chapter 1 – Muscle Chart

Knee

Muscle	Flexion	Extension	Internal rotation	External rotation
Vastus medialis		●		
Vastus lateralis		●		
Vastus intermedius		●		
Rectus femoris		●		
Sartorius	●			●
Semitendinosus	●		●	
Semimembranosus	●		●	
Biceps femoris	●			●
Gracilis	●		●	
Popliteus	●			
Gastrocnemius	●			

1 Seated Toe Extension

Part B — Innovations stretches

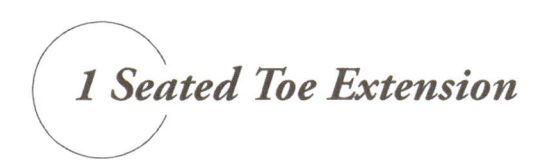

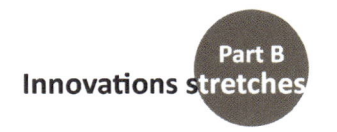

FLEXORS GROUP

HOW TO STRETCH: Photo A
- Clasp foot as pictured and bend toes backwards towards top of foot

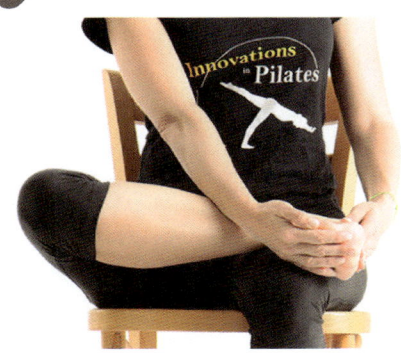

A

HOW TO CONTRACT: Photo B
- Press toes down into hand

HOW TO RESTRETCH: Photo B
- Bend toes further backwards
- Explore one toe at a time

B

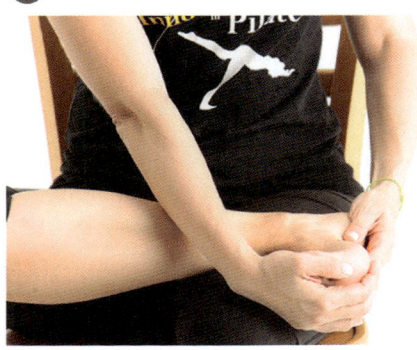

Major muscles stretched
- Intrinsic muscles of foot

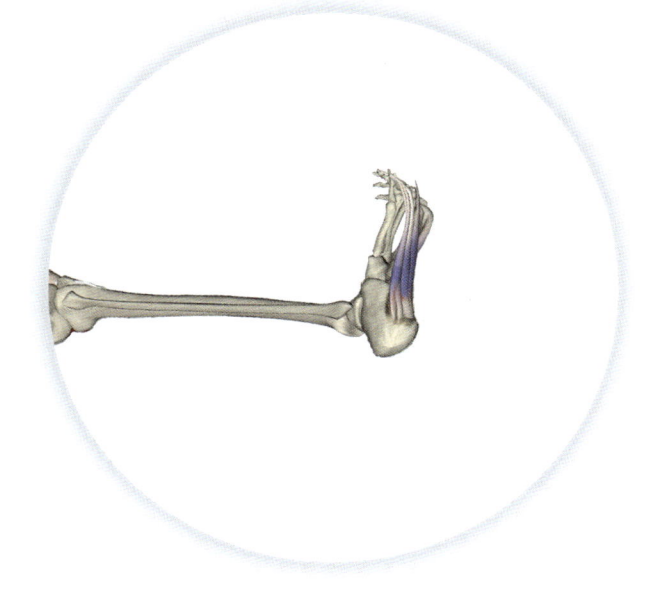

2 Standing Calf

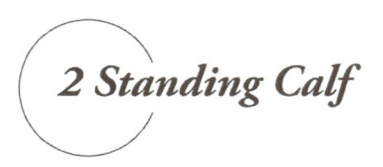

**Part B
Innovations stretches**

FLEXORS GROUP
HOW TO STRETCH: Photo A
- Secure box
- Take large step back and press rear heel into floor
- Lean hips forwards towards floor

HOW TO CONTRACT: Photo A
- Press ball of rear foot into floor

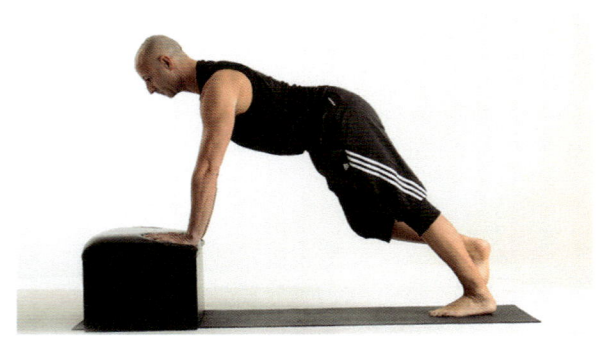

A

HOW TO RESTRETCH: Photo B
- Lower support or box, lean hips to floor
- Lift support leg so that weight-bearing is on stretch leg only

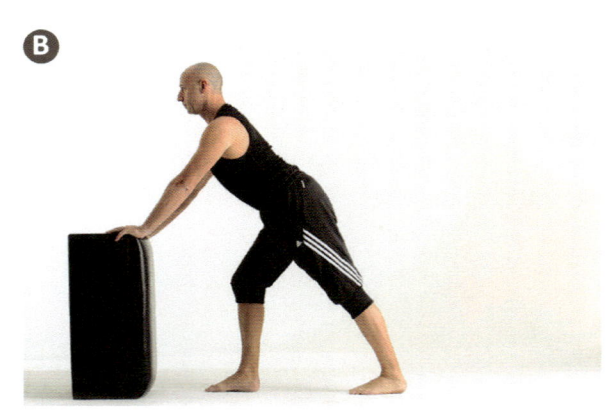

B

VARIATIONS - Photo C
- Turn leg inwards (medial rotation) to alter stretch sensations
- Turn leg outward (lateral rotation) to change stretch sensations (not shown)

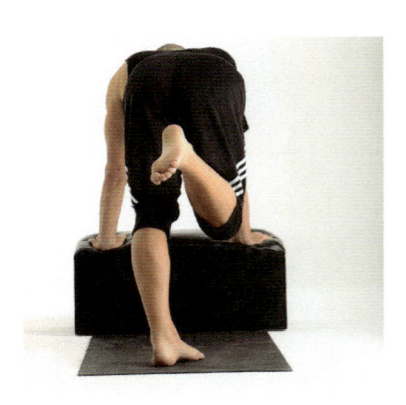

C

Photo D
- Bend stretch leg to emphasise soleus muscle

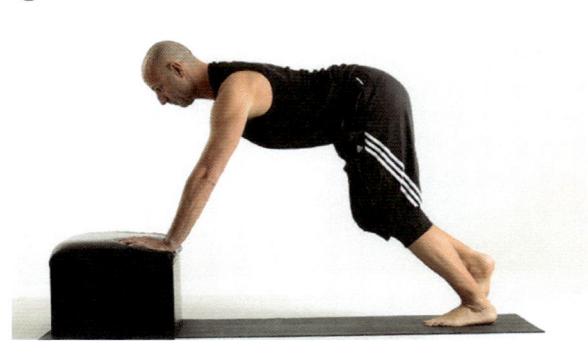

D

Major muscles stretched
- Soleus
- Gastrocnemius

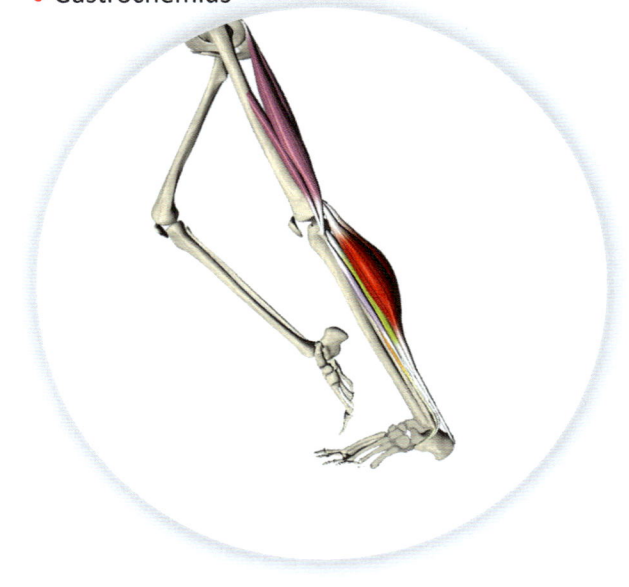

3 Lying Calf with Strap

Part B — Innovations stretches

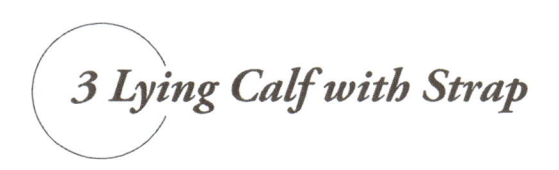

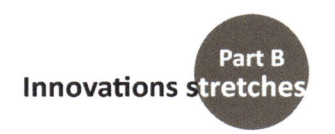

FLEXORS GROUP

HOW TO STRETCH: Photo A
- Place strap over ball of foot and pull downwards to point of tension

HOW TO CONTRACT: Photo A
- Press foot up into strap

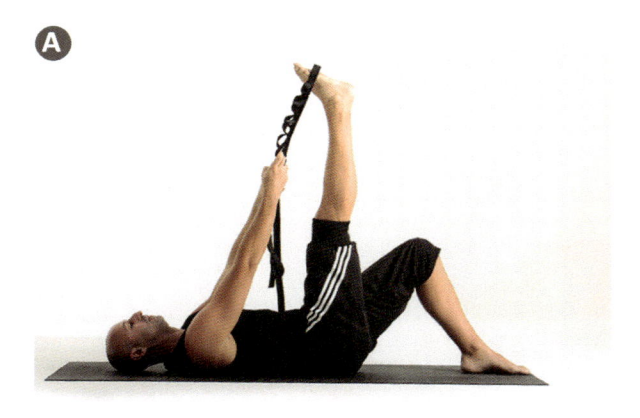

A

HOW TO RESTRETCH: Photo B
- Pull down on strap to restretch to new point of tension

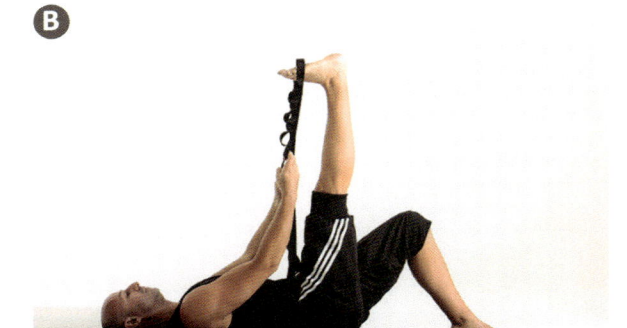

B

Major muscles stretched
- Soleus
- Gastrocnemius

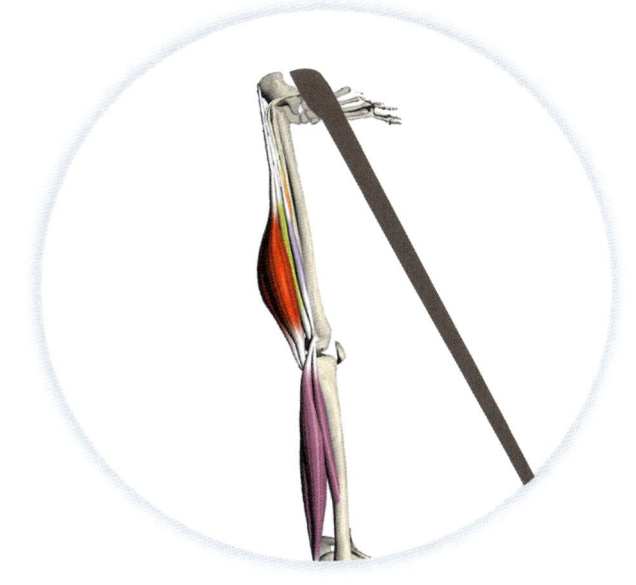

4 One Leg Dog Pose

Part B — Innovations stretches

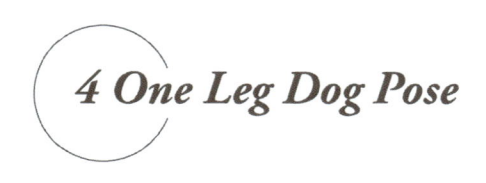

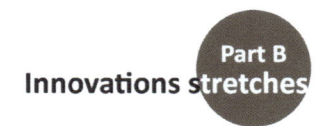

FLEXORS GROUP

HOW TO STRETCH: Photo A
- Secure your support or box
- Place weight on one leg
- Keep stance-leg straight
- Bend from hips to lower spine
- Lift chest to keep spine straight
- Align spine and arms

HOW TO CONTRACT: Photo A
- Press ball of rear foot into floor

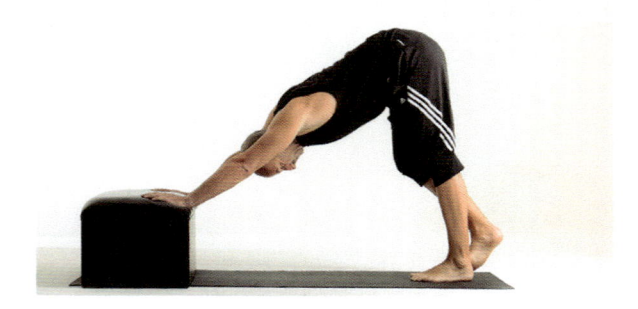

Ⓐ

HOW TO RESTRETCH: Photo B
- Lower hands to floor
- Align spine and arms
- Keep stance-leg straight

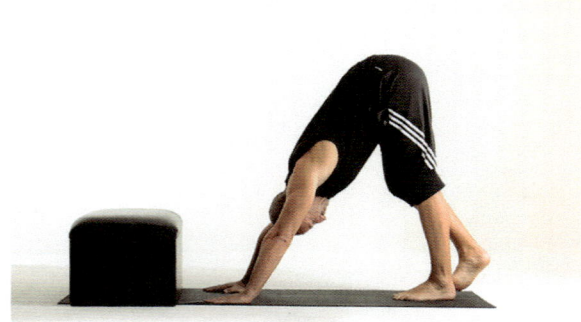

Ⓑ

ADVANCED VARIATION 1: Photo C
- Slowly raise non-stance leg
- Align leg with spine
- Partner to raise thigh of lifted leg

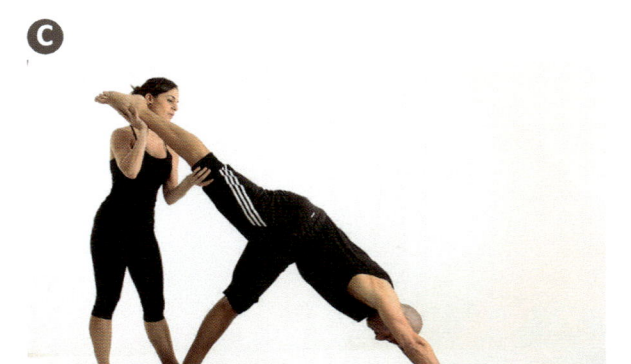

Ⓒ

HOW TO CONTRACT
- Press thigh of lifted leg down into partner

HOW TO RESTRETCH
- Lift thigh higher

Major muscles stretched
Soleus
- Hamstrings
- Gastrocnemius
Adductor magnus
Gluteus maximus

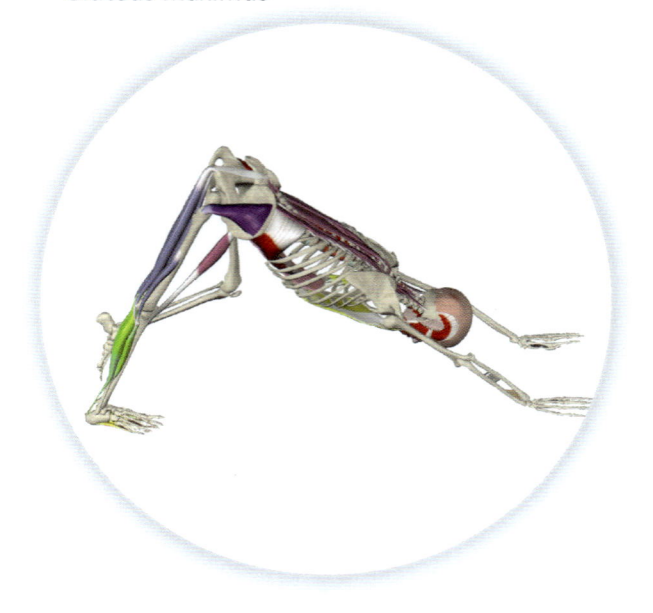

4 One Leg Dog Pose

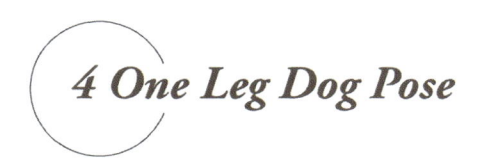

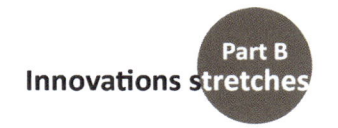

Part B — Innovations stretches

ADVANCED VARIATION 2

HOW TO STRETCH: Photo A
- Partner to raise thigh of lifted leg and bend knee, taking foot towards bottom

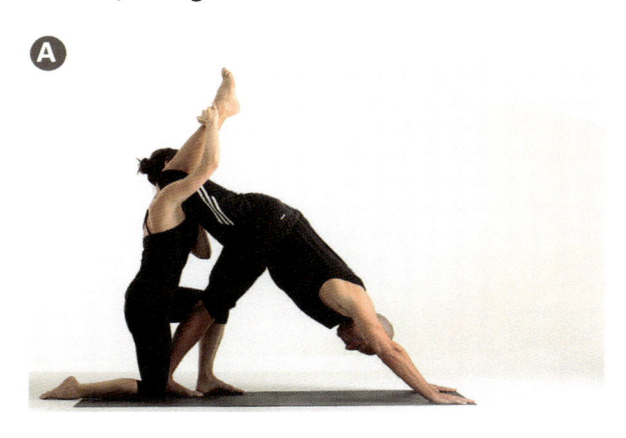

A

HOW TO CONTRACT: Photo B
- Press thigh of lifted leg down into partner
- Press foot of lifted leg into partner's hand

HOW TO RESTRETCH: Photo B
- Lift thigh and press foot towards bottom

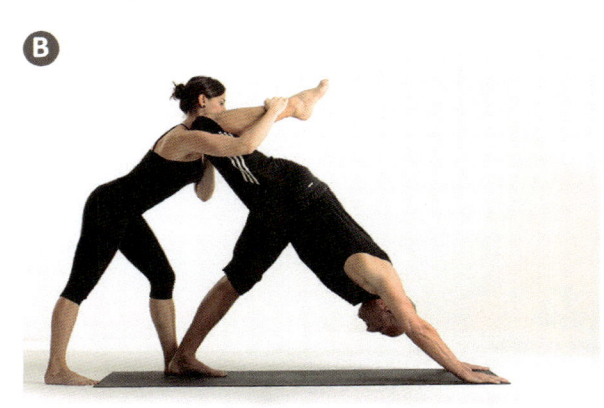

B

Major muscles stretched
- Hamstrings
- Quadriceps
- Hip flexors
- Calves
  Tibialis anterior

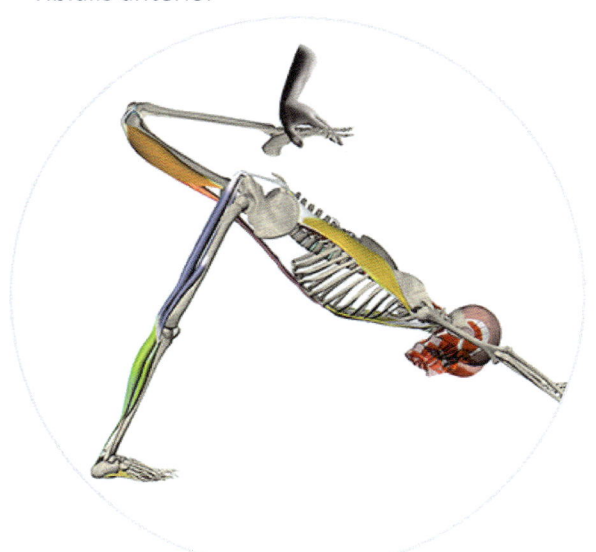

5 Toe Flexion

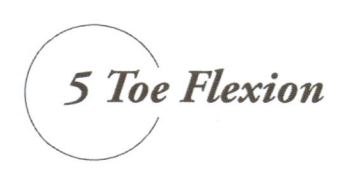

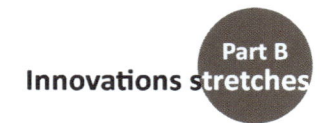

Part B — Innovations stretches

EXTENSORS AND DORSIFLEXORS

HOW TO STRETCH: Photo A
- Clasp ankle and foot as pictured
- Stabilise ankle
- Press toes and top of forefoot down

HOW TO CONTRACT: Photo A
- Press toes up into hand

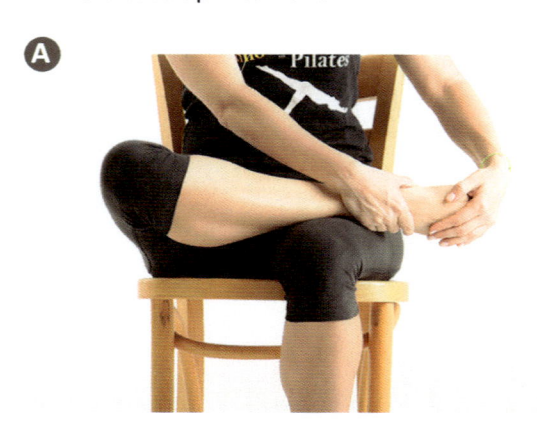

Ⓐ

HOW TO RESTRETCH: Photo B
- Bend toes further downwards towards sole of foot
- Explore one toe at a time

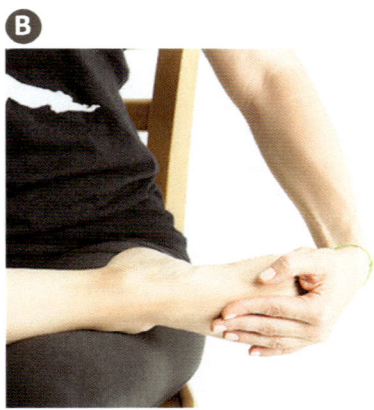

Ⓑ

Major muscles stretched
- Tibialis anterior
  Extensor hallucis
- Extensor digitorum

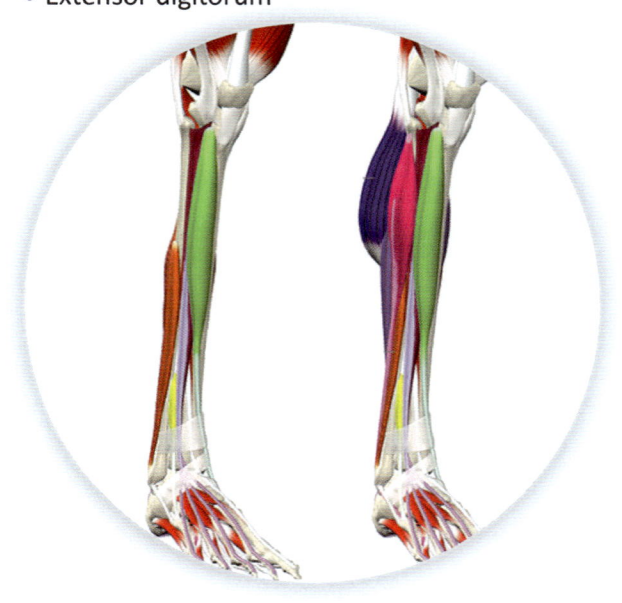

6 Seated Tibialis Anterior

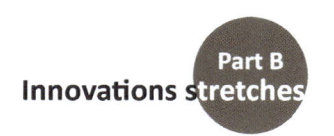

**Part B
Innovations stretches**

EXTENSORS AND DORSIFLEXORS

HOW TO STRETCH: Photo A
- Clasp foot as pictured and bend foot downward

HOW TO CONTRACT: Photo A
- Press foot up into hand

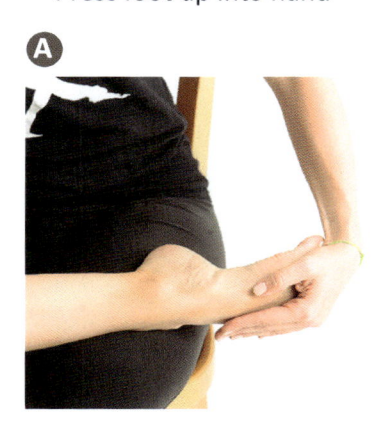

A

HOW TO RESTRETCH: Photo B
- Bend foot and toes further downward
- Explore one toe at a time

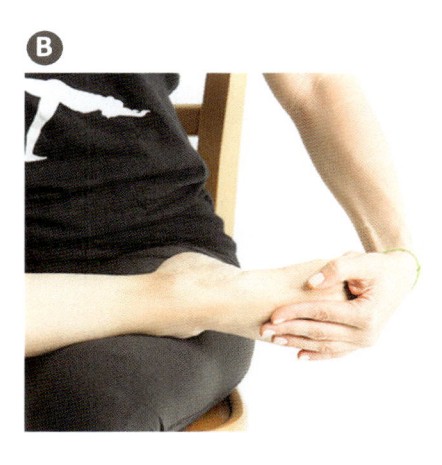

B

Major muscles stretched
- Tibialis anterior
  Extensor hallicus
- Extensor digitorum

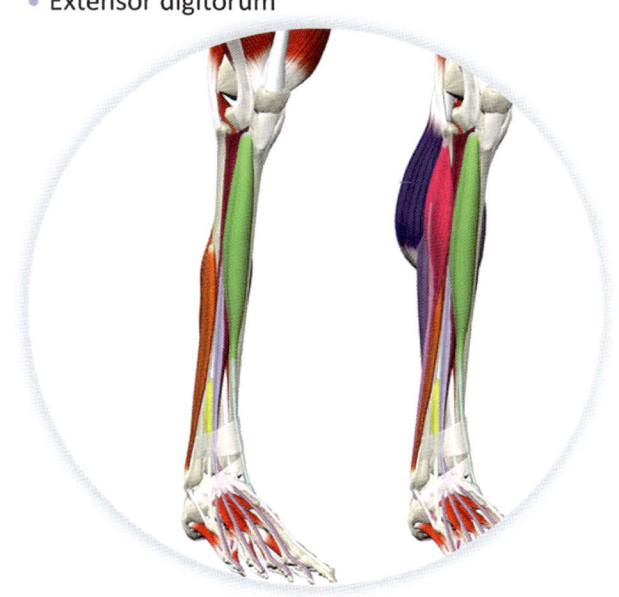

7 Floor Tibialis Anterior

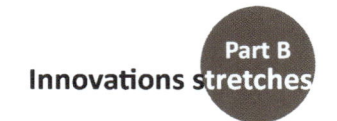

Part B
Innovations stretches

EXTENSORS AND DORSIFLEXORS
HOW TO STRETCH: Photo A
- Sit on feet as pictured

HOW TO CONTRACT: Photo A
- Press top of feet into floor

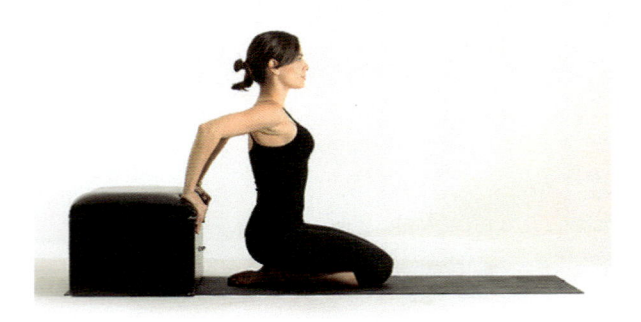

A

HOW TO RESTRETCH: Photo B
- Roll pelvis back

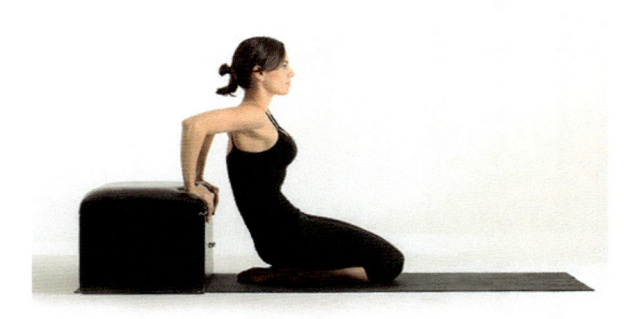

B

Photo C
- Emphasise one leg
- Lift knee higher from floor

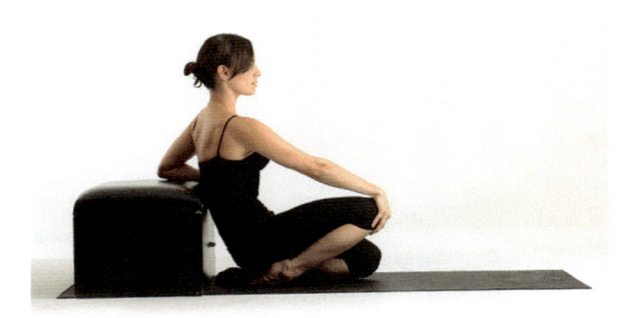

C

Major muscles stretched
- Tibialis anterior
  Extensor hallicus
- Extensor digitorum

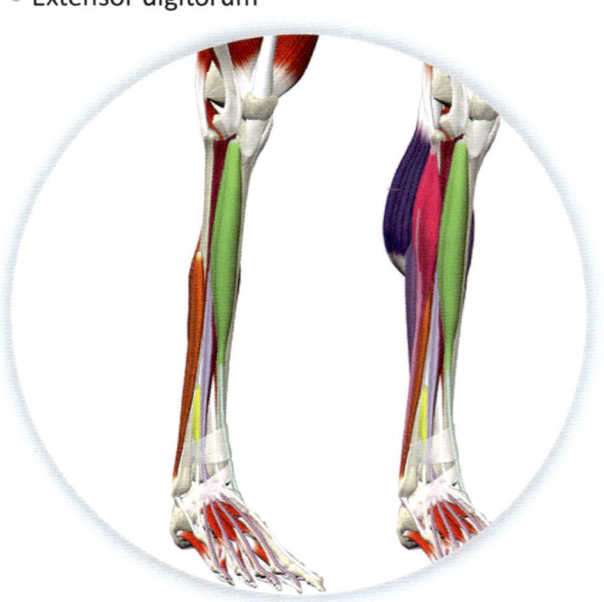

8 Seated Inversion

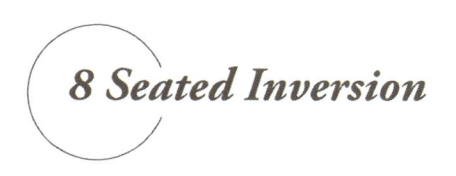

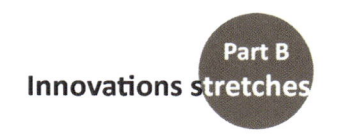

Part B — Innovations stretches

INVERTERS

HOW TO STRETCH: Photo A
- Clasp foot as pictured
- Turn sole of foot inwards

HOW TO CONTRACT: Photo A
- Press foot back towards pre-stretch position

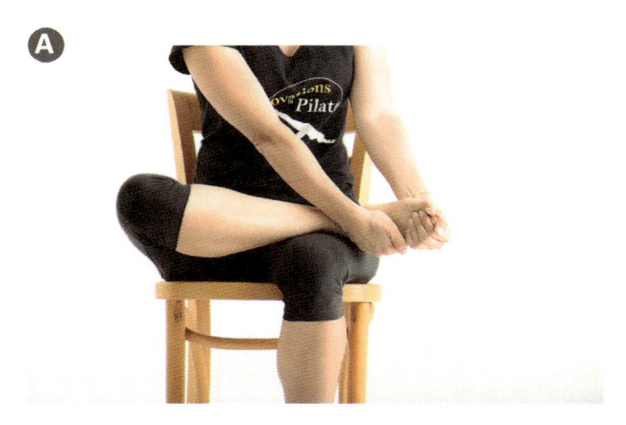

A

HOW TO RESTRETCH: Photo B
- Turn sole of foot further inward

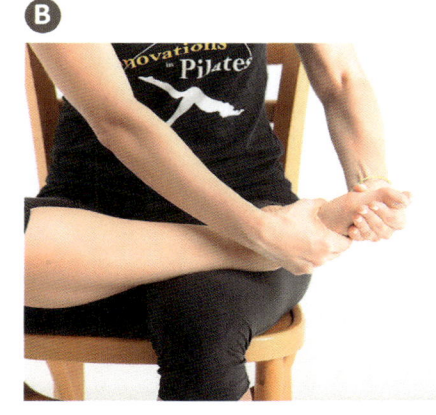

B

Major muscles stretched
- Peroneus longus
- Peroneus brevis
- Peroneus tertius

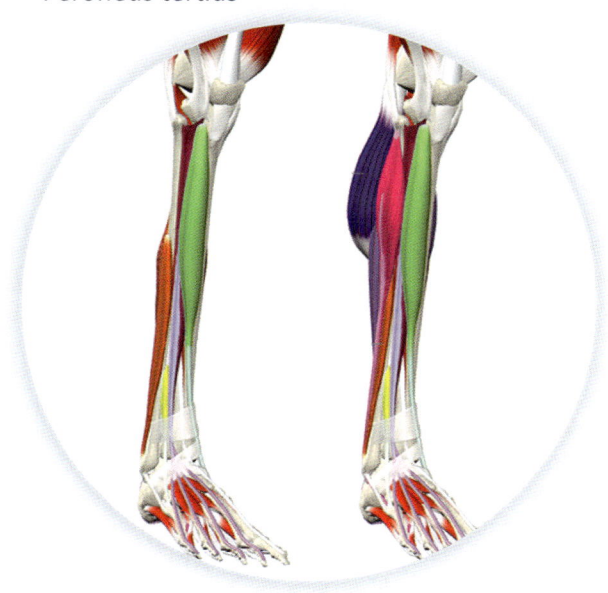

9 Inversion with Strap

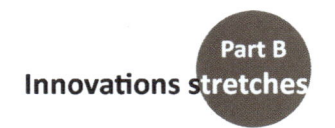

Part B — Innovations stretches

INVERTERS

HOW TO STRETCH: Photo A
- Place strap on forefoot and gently turn foot inwards

HOW TO CONTRACT: Photo A
- Push sole of foot towards ceiling

A

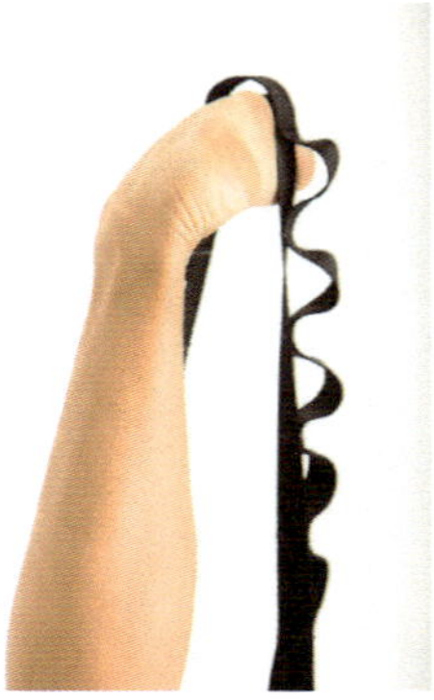

HOW TO RESTRETCH: Photo B
- Pull down on strap to new point of tension

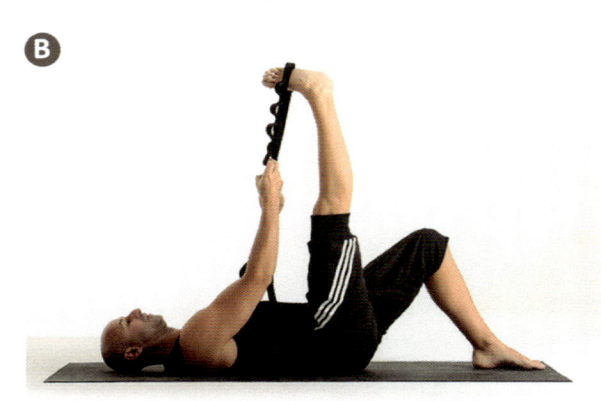

B

Major muscles stretched
- Peroneus longus
- Peroneus brevis
- Peroneus tertius

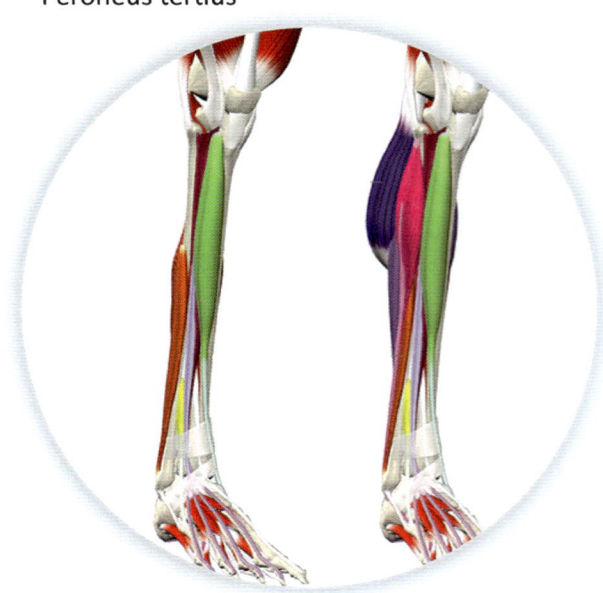

10 Seated Eversion

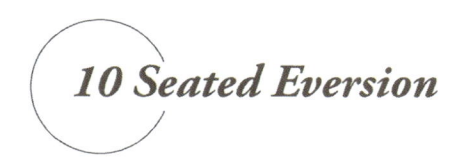

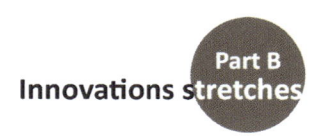

Part B
Innovations stretches

INVERTERS

HOW TO STRETCH: Photo A
- Clasp foot as pictured and turn sole of foot outwards, away from centre

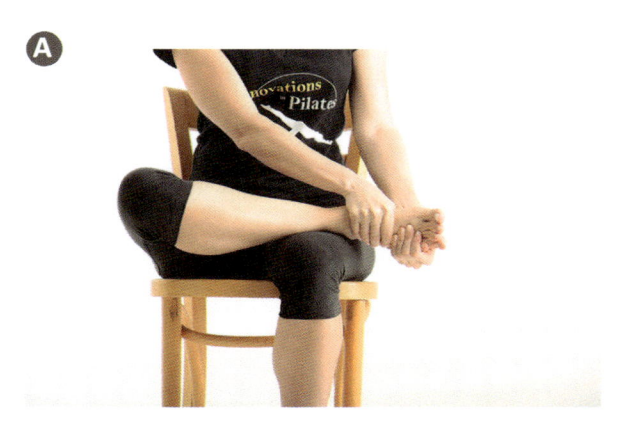

HOW TO CONTRACT: Photo B
- Press sole of foot back towards centre

HOW TO RESTRETCH: Photo B
- Twist sole of foot further away from centre/neutral position

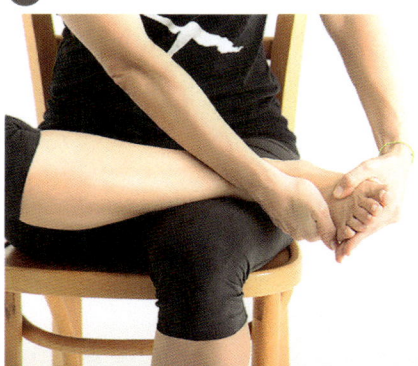

Major muscles stretched
- Tibialis posterior
  Flexor digitorum longus
- Flexor hallucis longus

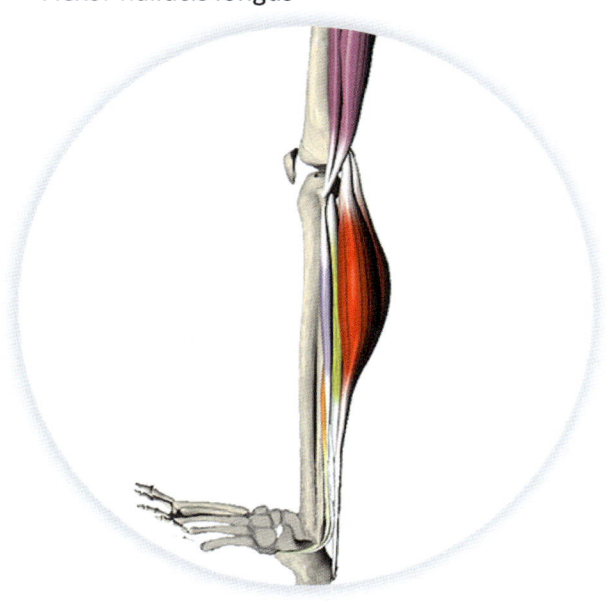

11 Eversion with Strap

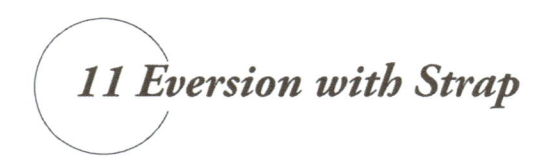

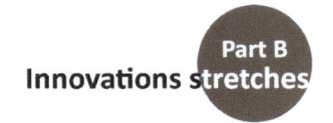

Innovations stretches — Part B

INVERTERS

HOW TO STRETCH: Photo A
- Place strap over ball of foot and pull to turn sole of foot outwards from centre

HOW TO CONTRACT: Photo A
- Press sole of foot back towards centre

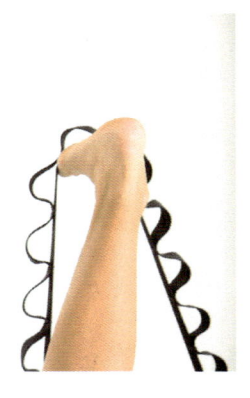

A

HOW TO RESTRETCH: Photo B
- Pull on outside of strap to turn sole of foot further from centre

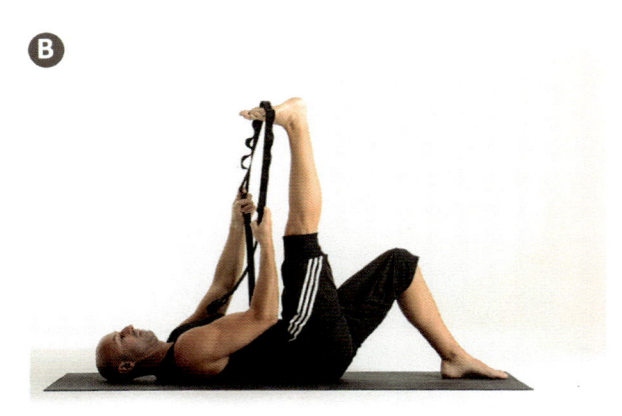

B

Major muscles stretched
- Tibialis posterior
  Flexor digitorum longus
- Flexor hallucis longus

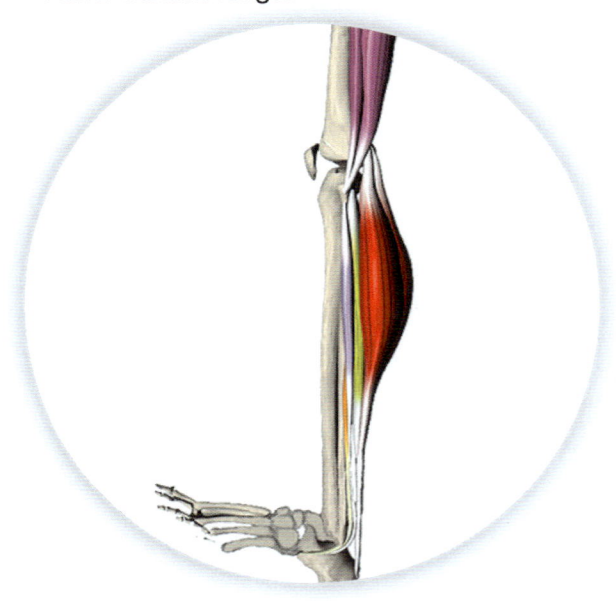

The Hamstrings
Chapter 2

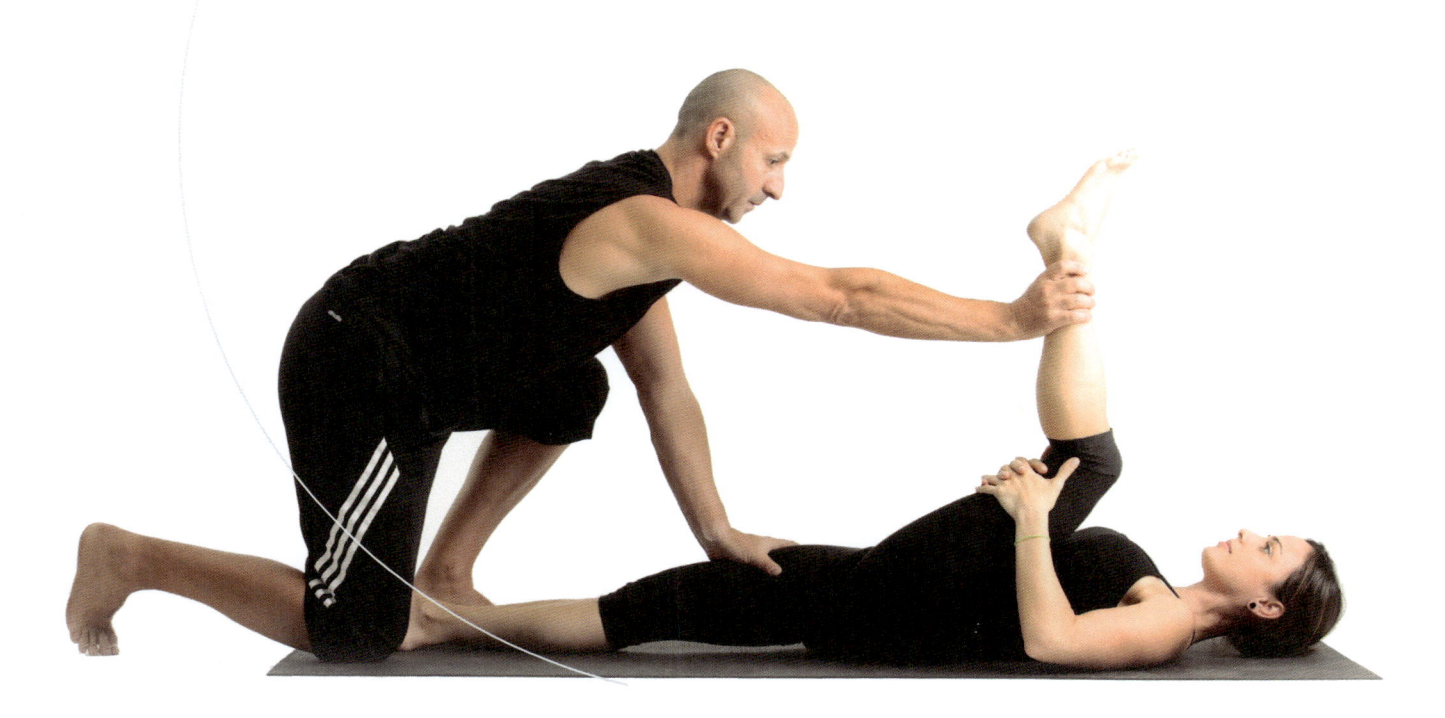

Chapter 2 – Muscle Chart

Hip

Muscle	Flexion	Extension	Adduction	Abduction	Internal rotation	External rotation
Gluteus maximus		●				●
Gluteus medius	●	●		●	●	●
Gluteus minumus	●	●		●	●	●
Tensor fascia lata	●			●	●	
Psoas major	●					●
Iliacus	●					●
Rectus femoris	●			●		
Sartorius	●			●		●
Pectineus	●		●			●
Adductor magnus		●	●			●
Adductor longus	●		●			●
Adductor brevis	●		●			●
Gracilis	●		●			●
Piriformis				●		●
Gemellus superior				●		●
Gemellus inferior				●		●
Obturator internus				●		●
Obturator externus						●
Quadratus femoris			●		●	●
Semitendinosus		●			●	
Semimembranosus		●				
Biceps femoris		●				●

Knee

Muscle	Flexion	Extension	Internal rotation	External rotation
Vastus medialis		●		
Vastus lateralis		●		
Vastus intermedius		●		
Rectus femoris		●		
Sartorius	●			●
Semitendinosus	●		●	
Semimembranosus	●		●	
Biceps femoris	●			●
Gracilis	●		●	
Popliteus	●			
Gastrocnemius	●			

12 Foam Roller Hamstring

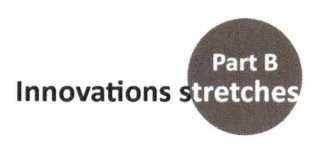

Part B — Innovations stretches

HOW TO STRETCH: Photo A
- Sit as pictured and pull chest towards thighs
- Slowly straighten legs keeping chest in contact with thighs

HOW TO CONTRACT: Photo A
- Press the ankles or feet down into the roller

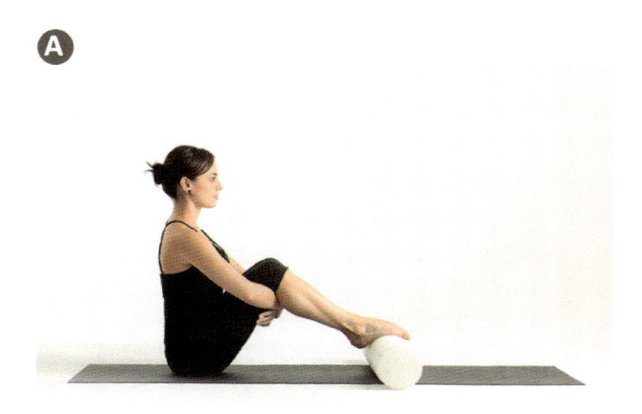

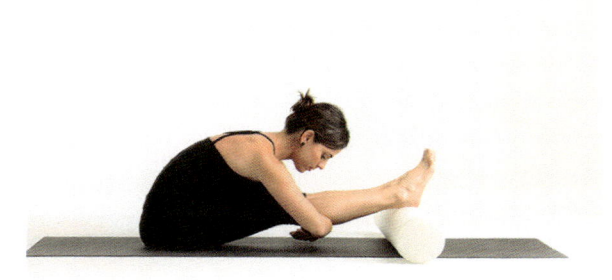

A

HOW TO RESTRETCH: Photo B
- Straighten the legs further, keeping chest on legs

HOW TO INTENSIFY: Photo B
- Bend toes further backwards
- Lift chest to straighten spine

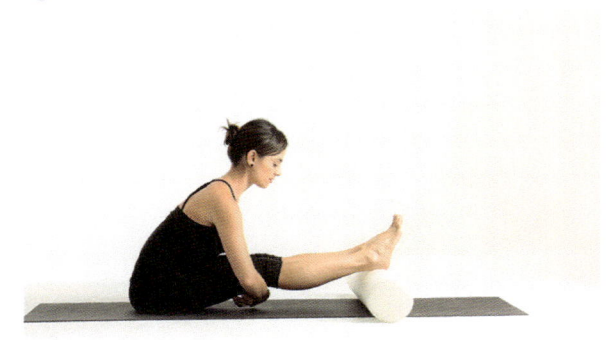

B

FOR THE SPINE: Photo C
- Allow back to bend/flex, pull chest closer to legs

C

Major muscles stretched
- Erector spinae
- Hamstrings
- Calves
  Adductor magnus
- Gluteus maximus

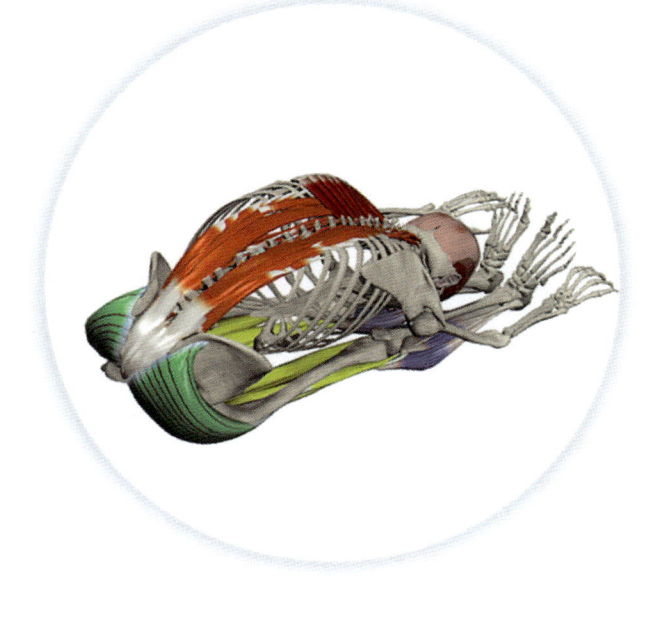

13 Hamstring Glute Exploration

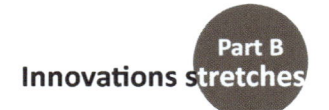

Part B Innovations stretches

HOW TO STRETCH: Photos A, B, C, D
- Allow body to fold at waist and drop slowly towards floor
- Allow head to drop also
- Turn slowly to one side and bend the opposite knee; for example, hand and arms over right leg and bend left knee. Repeat for other side

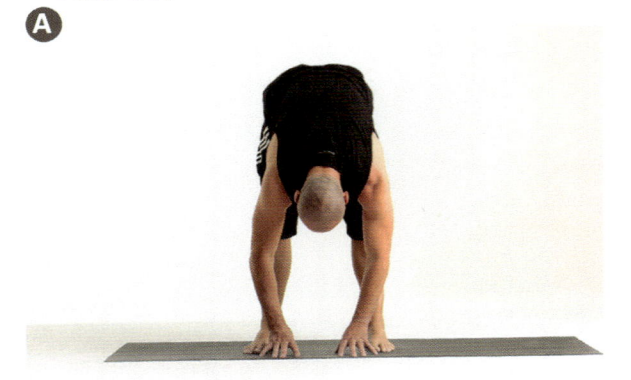

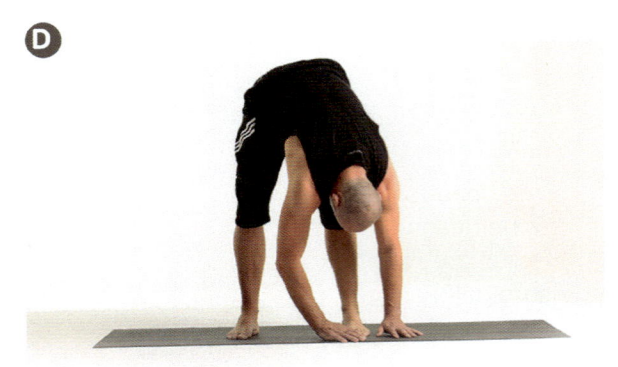

A

B

C

D

HOW TO CONTRACT: Photo E
- Clasp both ankles and arch your back as if to straighten the spine. Hold for five breaths.

HOW TO RESTRETCH: Photo E
- Keep spine straight and pull chest down between legs. Hold for ten breaths

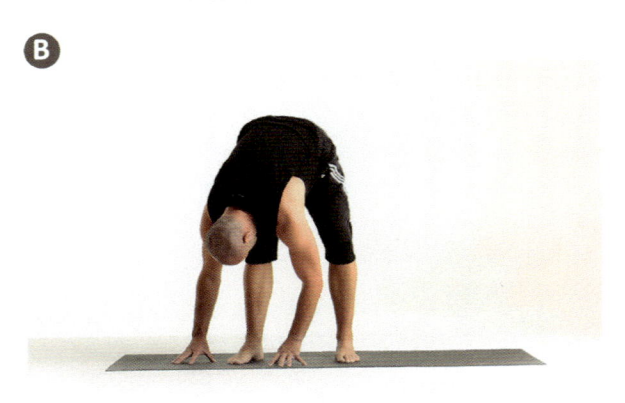

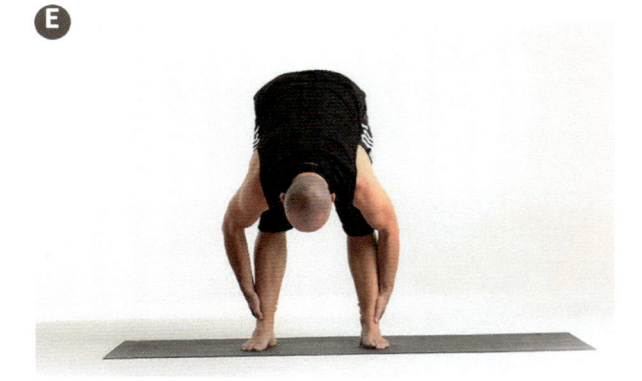

E

Major muscles stretched

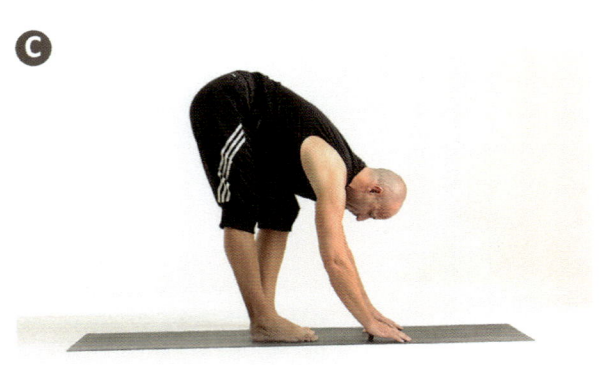

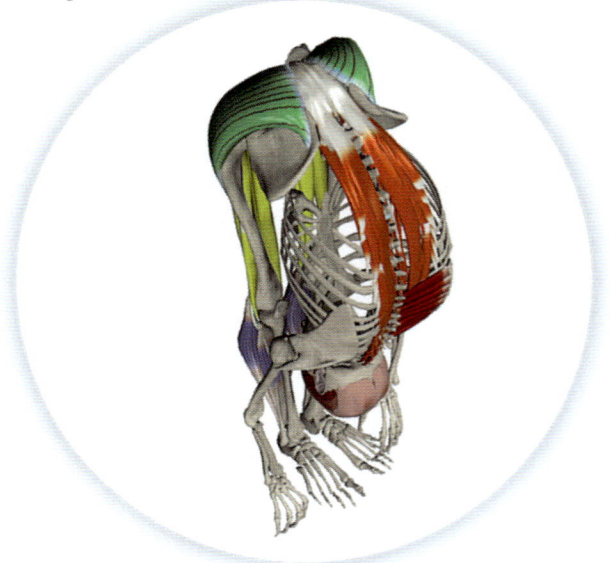

- Erector spinae
- Hamstrings
- Calves
- Glutes
- Adductor magnus

14 Hamstring Glute Partner

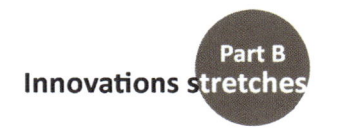

Part B Innovations stretches

HOW TO STRETCH: Photo A
- Lie as pictured, with partner using straight arms to move and support you
- Pull one leg back towards your chest or armpit and hook arm around hamstrings
- Partner leans towards you, opening out angle at your knee joint
- do not allow thigh to creep away from chest

HOW TO CONTRACT: Photo B
- Press thigh away from chest while simultaneously pressing heel towards bottom

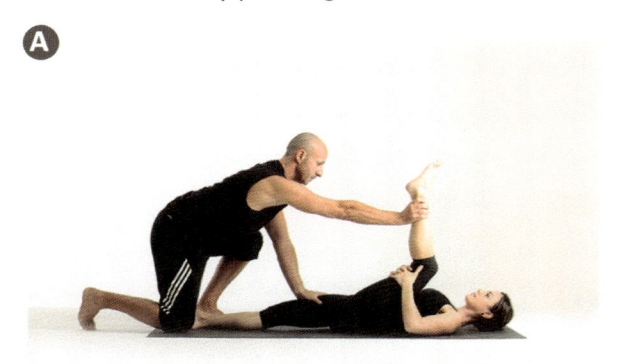

A

HOW TO RESTRETCH: Photo B
- Pull thigh as close as possible to chest or armpit and open the ankle further at the knee joint

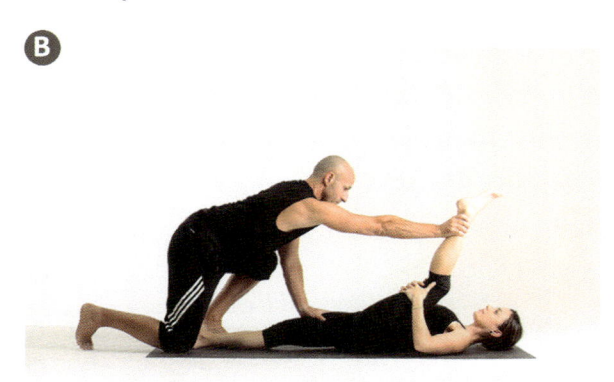

B

Major muscles stretched
- Gluteus maximus
- Hamstrings
  Adductor magnus
- Rectus femoris
- TFL
- Iliopsoas

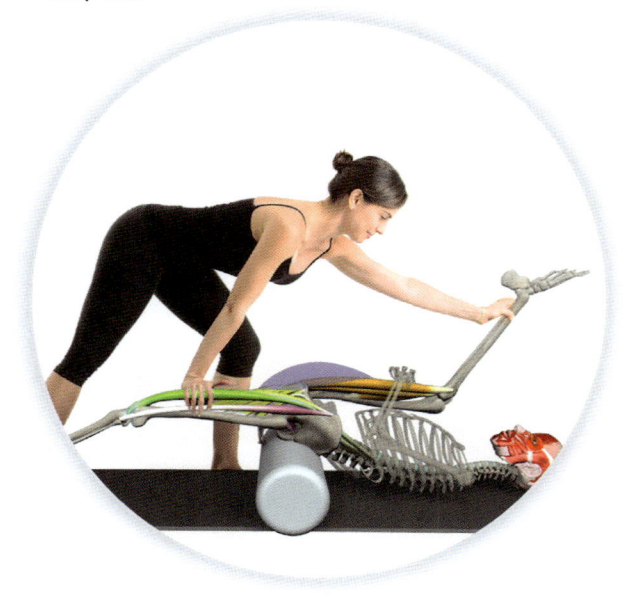

15 Lying Medial and Lateral

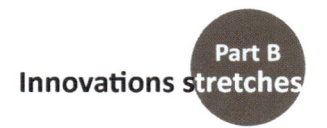

Part B Innovations stretches

HOW TO STRETCH: Photo A
- Place foot into strap and raise leg to point of tension
- Keeping both hips on floor, take leg towards or across midline of body to stretch biceps femoris
- Keep knee firm and straight

HOW TO CONTRACT: Photo A
- Press leg away from midline of body

HOW TO RESTRETCH: Photo A
- Take leg further across midline of body and also towards shoulder (greater hip flexion) for piriformis emphasis

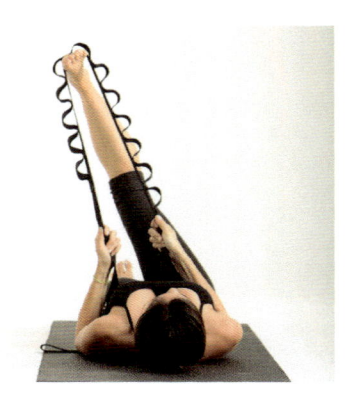

HOW TO CONTRACT: Photo B
- Press leg back towards midline

HOW TO RESTRETCH: Photo C
- Take leg further from midline of body
- Bend opposite knee to counterbalance if required

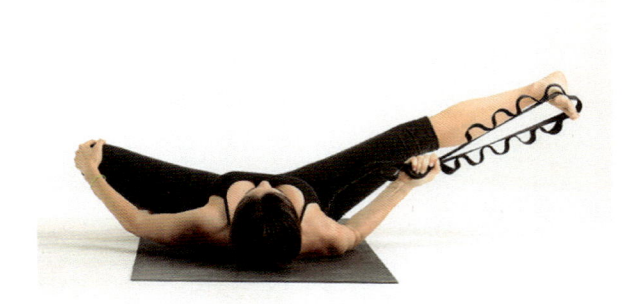

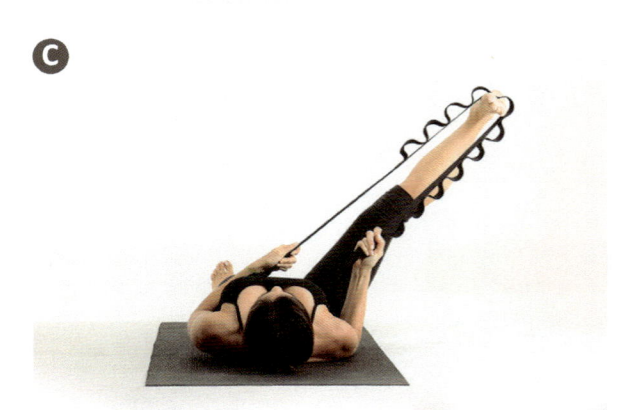

- Biceps Femoris
- Piriformis

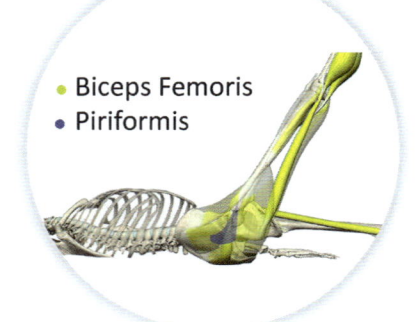

MEDIAL HAMSTRINGS/ADDUCTORS
HOW TO STRETCH: Photo B
- Take leg towards chest until point of tension
- Take leg away from midline of body to stretch medial hamstrings and adductors
- Keep both hips on floor

Major muscles stretched

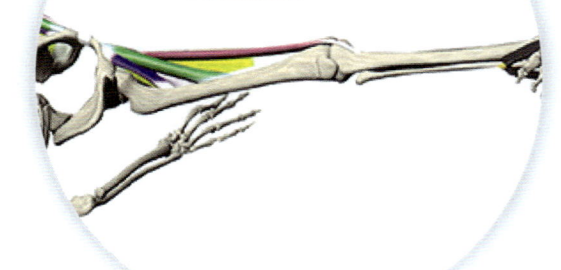

- Adductors magnus
- Adductors longus
- Gracilis
- Pectineus

16 Lying Straight Leg Hamstring

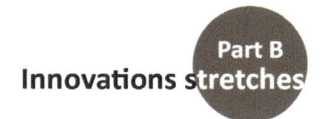

**Part B
Innovations stretches**

HOW TO STRETCH: Photo A
- Place strap across foot and pull leg to point of tension
- Keep knee straight and firm

HOW TO CONTRACT: Photo A
- Press entire leg towards floor

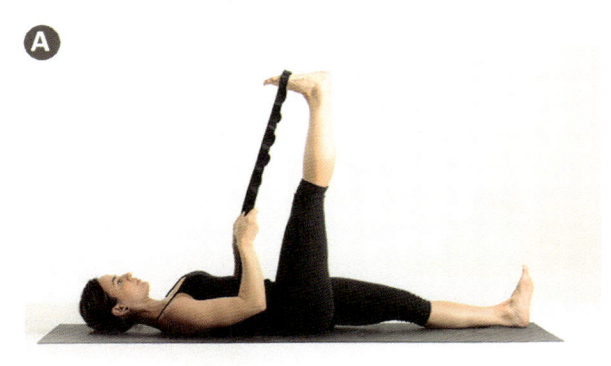

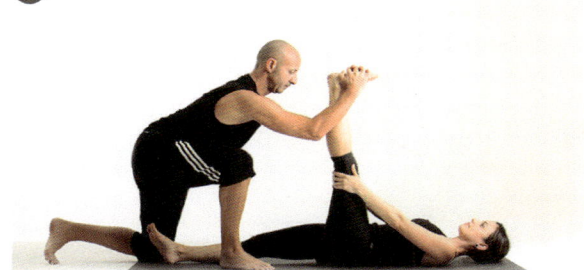

A

HOW TO RESTRETCH: Photo B
- Contract quads and pull leg towards chest

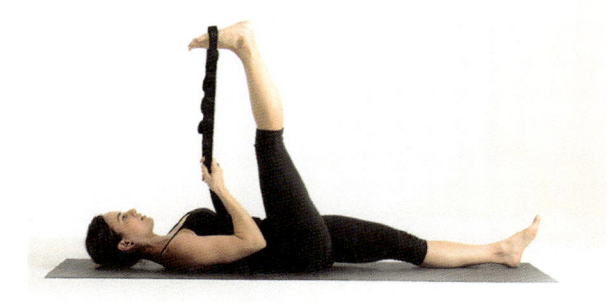

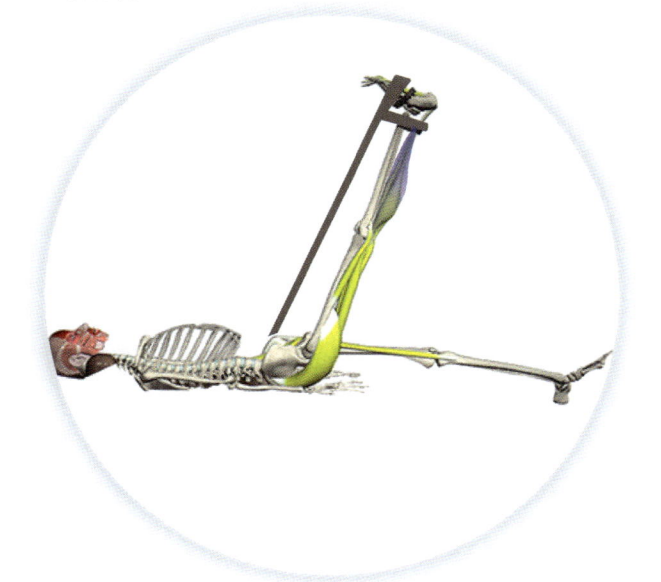

B

PARTNER ASSISTANCE: Photo C
- Partner must be secure, with straight arms
- Place hands as pictured and keep knee straight while pressing leg towards chest/armpit
- Contractions as in solo version

C

VARIATION: Photo D
- Press ball of foot down to accentuate calf and back of knee

D

Major muscles stretched
- Hamstrings
- Calves

17 The Mex Stretch

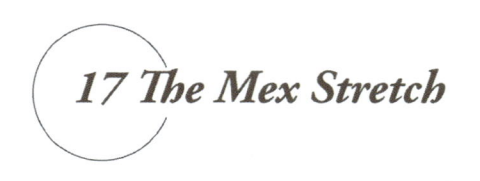

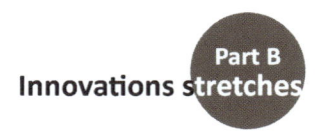

Part B — Innovations stretches

HOW TO STRETCH: Photo A
- Sit as pictured and turn legs outwards
- Slowly try to straighten legs, keeping spine straight

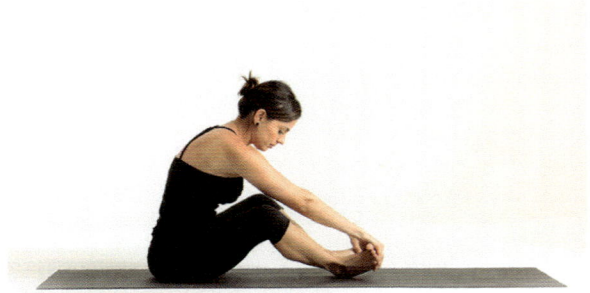

A

HOW TO CONTRACT: Photo B
- Lift chest to straighten spine
- Press heels into floor, then into each other

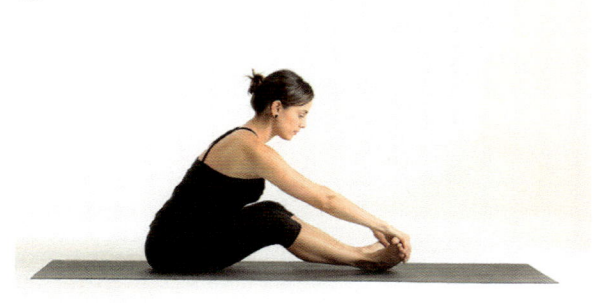

B

HOW TO RESTRETCH: Photo C
- Slowly straighten legs with spine straight

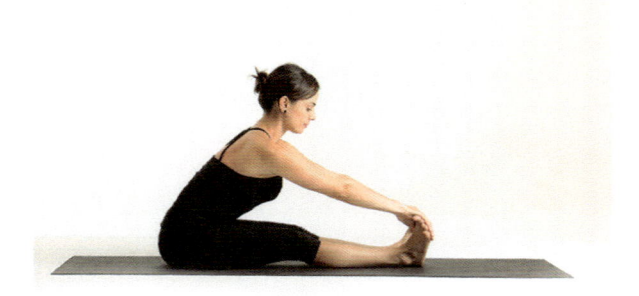

C

Major muscles stretched
- Hamstrings
- Calves

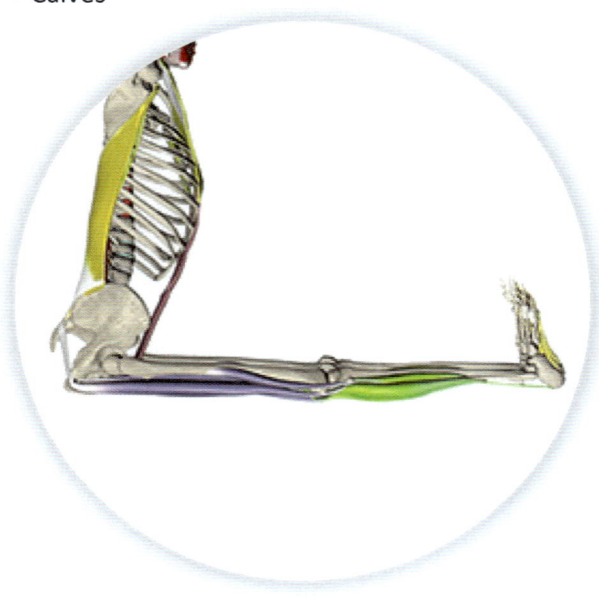

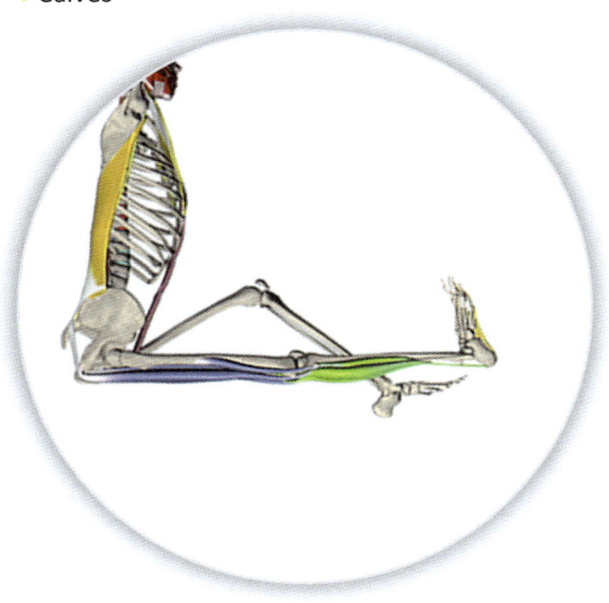

18 Seated Bent-Leg Hamstring

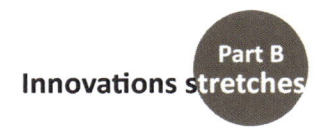

**Part B
Innovations stretches**

HOW TO STRETCH: Photo A
- Place strap over foot and lift chest
- Try to straighten leg to point of tension

HOW TO CONTRACT: Photo A
- Press heel into floor

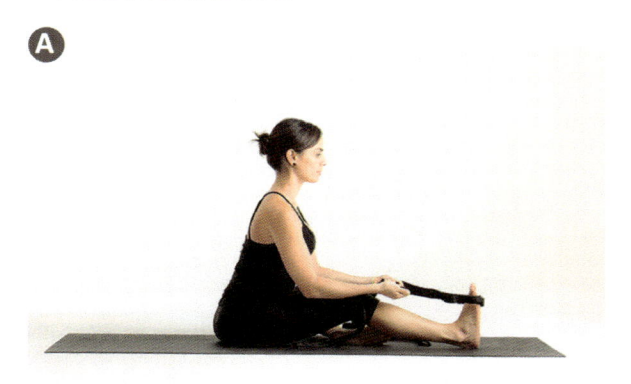

A

HOW TO RESTRETCH: Photo B
- Lift chest to straighten spine
- Try to straighten leg fully by sliding heel away

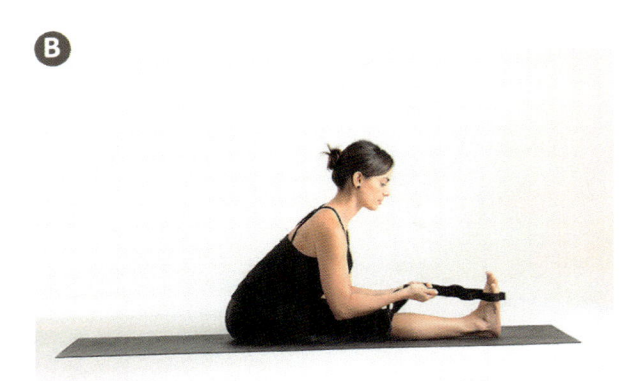

B

Major muscles stretched
- Hamstrings
- Calves

19 Seated Calf, Hamstring Partner

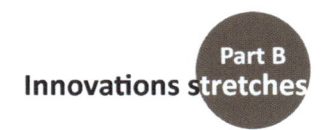

Part B
Innovations stretches

HOW TO STRETCH: Photo A
- Sit as pictured with one leg bent
- Place strap over straight leg
- Keeping spine straight, bend forwards at hip
- Partner to press into sacrum to assist with forwards bend and maintaining neutral spine/ anterior tilt

HOW TO CONTRACT: Photo A
- Press foot/heel into floor

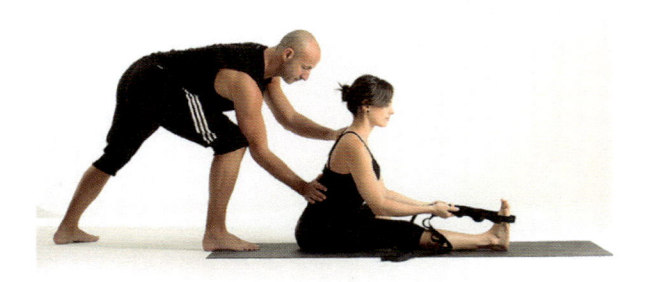

A

HOW TO RESTRETCH: Photo B
- Lean chest towards leg, keeping spine straight
- Partner to assist with lean
- Pull on strap for calf emphasis

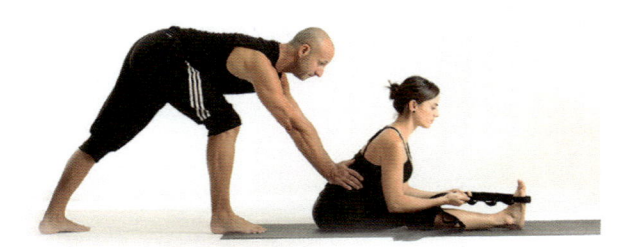

B

Major muscles stretched
- Hamstrings
- Calves

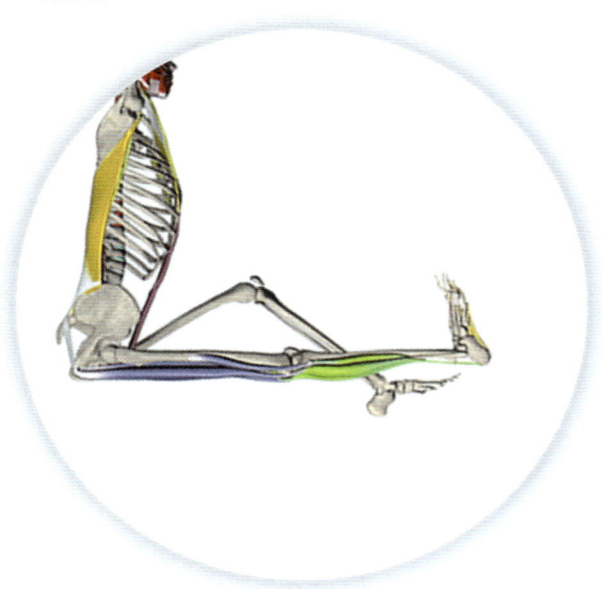

The Hip Flexors and Quadriceps

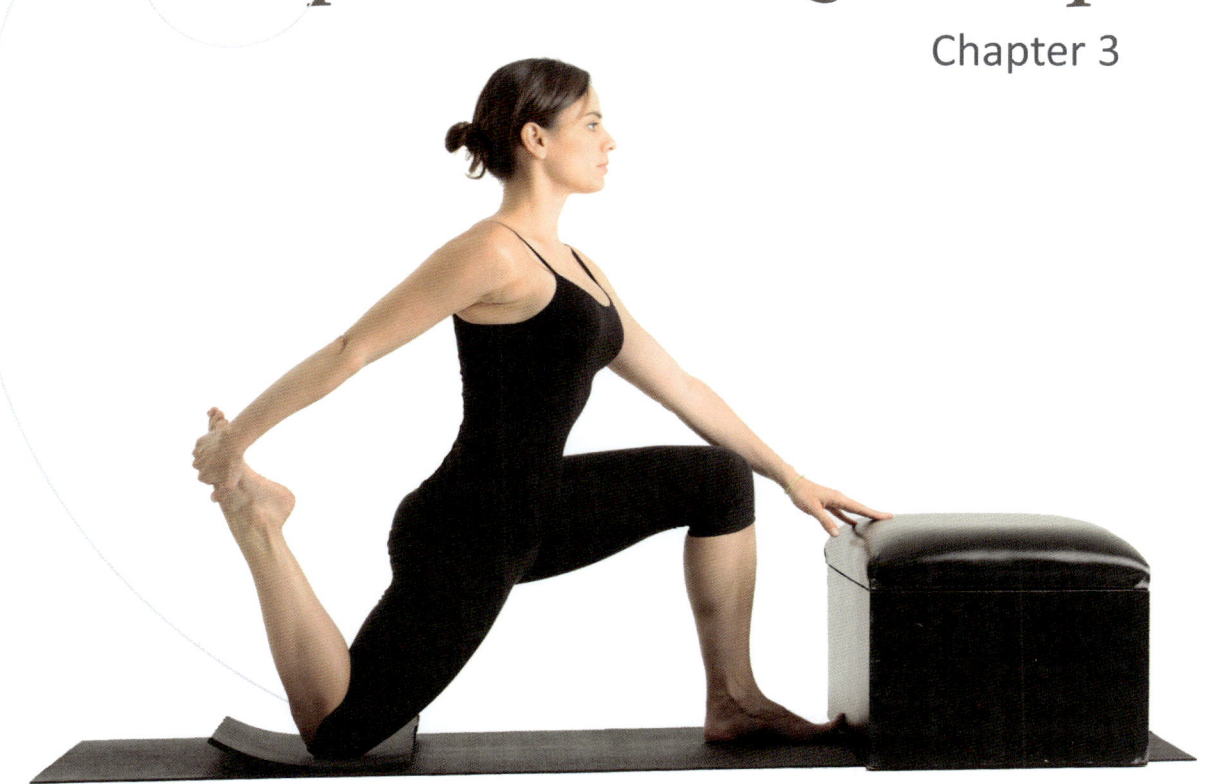

Chapter 3

Chapter 3 – Muscle Chart

Hip

Muscle	Flexion	Extension	Adduction	Abduction	Internal rotation	External rotation
Gluteus maximus		●				●
Gluteus medius	●	●		●	●	●
Gluteus minumus	●	●		●	●	●
Tensor fascia lata	●			●	●	
Psoas major	●					●
Iliacus	●					●
Rectus femoris	●			●		
Sartorius	●			●		●
Pectineus	●		●			
Adductor magnus		●	●			●
Adductor longus	●		●			●
Adductor brevis	●		●			●
Gracilis	●		●			●
Piriformis				●		●
Gemellus superior				●		●
Gemellus inferior				●		●
Obturator internus				●		●
Obturator externus						●
Quadratus femoris			●		●	●
Semitendinosus		●			●	
Semimembranosus		●				
Biceps femoris		●				●

Knee

Muscle	Flexion	Extension	Internal rotation	External rotation
Vastus medialis		●		
Vastus lateralis		●		
Vastus intermedius		●		
Rectus femoris		●		
Sartorius	●			●
Semitendinosus	●		●	
Semimembranosus	●		●	
Biceps femoris	●			●
Gracilis	●		●	
Popliteus	●			
Gastrocnemius	●			

20 Foam Roller Hamstrings Glute

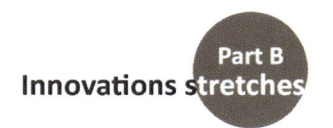

Part B
Innovations stretches

HOW TO STRETCH: Photo A
- Lift hips from lying position and place roller under sacrum
- Clasp thigh and pull towards chest
- Partner places hands as pictured and leans onto both legs

HOW TO CONTRACT: Photo A
- Press both legs into partner's hands

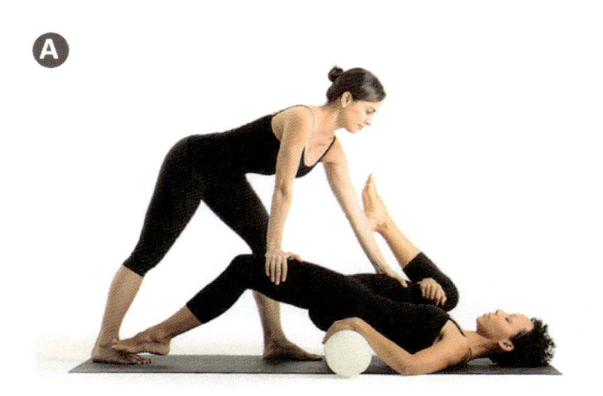

A

HOW TO RESTRETCH: Photo B
- Shift grip onto ankle and open out knee joint to point of tension
- Person being stretched holds top thigh onto chest

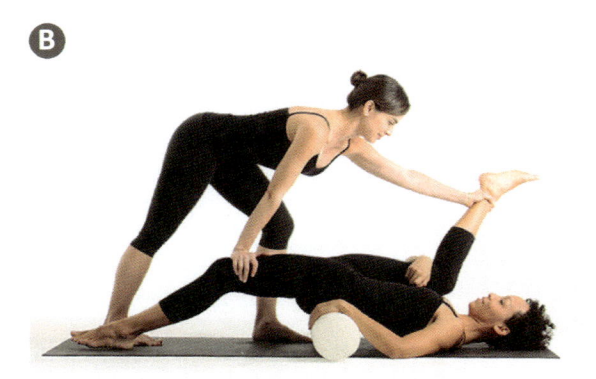

B

Major muscles stretched
- Iliopsoas
- Hamstring
- Adductors magnus
  Gluteus maximus
- TFL
- Rectus femoris

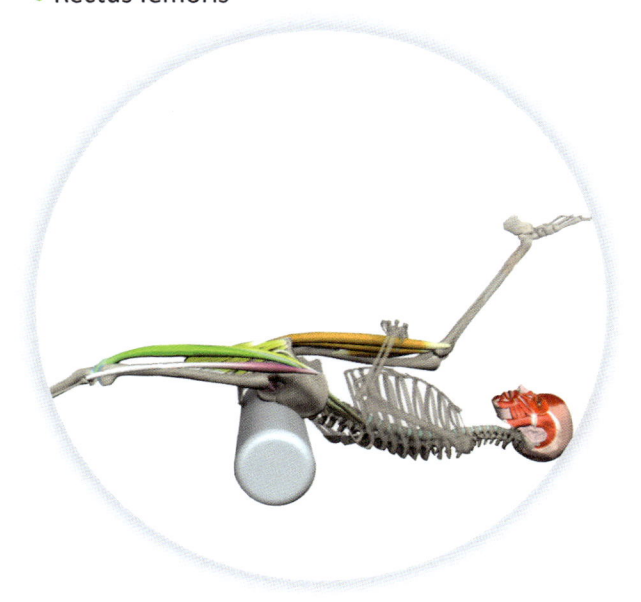

21 Kneeling Quadriceps Box

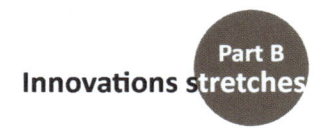

Part B
Innovations stretches

HOW TO STRETCH: Photo A
- Sit in front of secure box with elbows bent
- Shift weight onto arms
- Sit onto heels

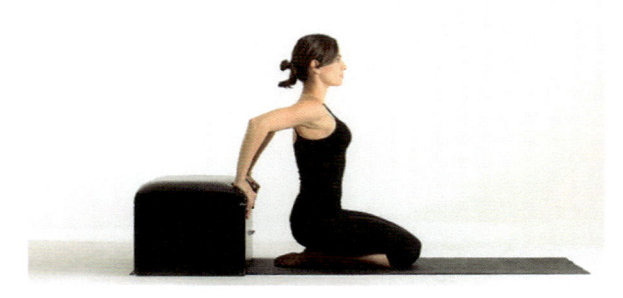

A

HOW TO CONTRACT: Photo B
- Roll pelvis posteriorly
- Bend elbows as required to point of tension
- Keep knees on floor
- Keep legs parallel
- Press shins and feet into floor

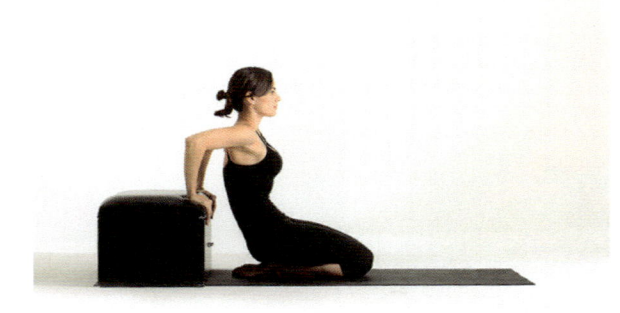

B

HOW TO RESTRETCH: Photo C
- Tilt pelvis further and drop slowly onto elbows if possible
- Tighten and scoop abdominals to prevent lumbar extension/arching

C

Photo D
- Partner to press on thighs and keep legs aligned
- To contract further, press thighs up into partner's hands

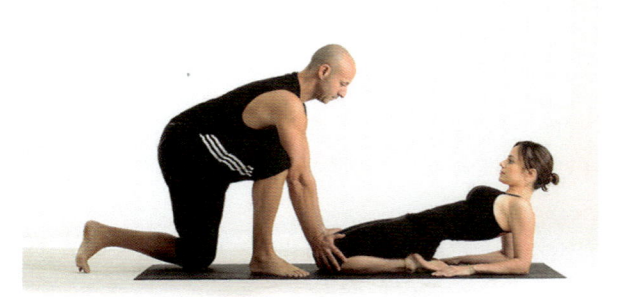

D

Photo E
- Partner places toes onto knees to anchor thighs to floor
- To restretch, roll pelvis further posteriorly and lean away from partner

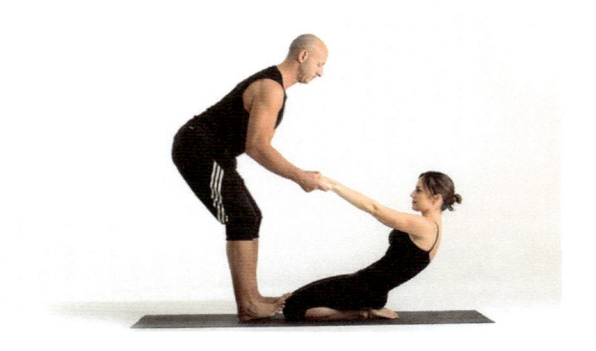

E

Major muscles stretched
Quadriceps
Rectus femoris
Tibialis anterior

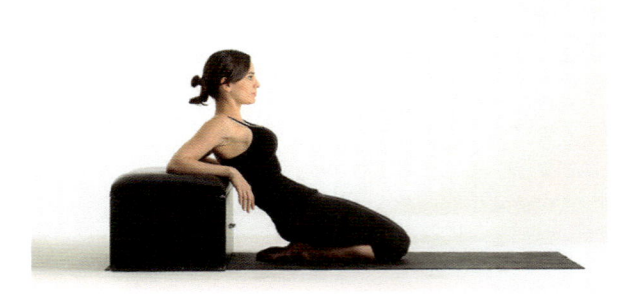

22 Kneeling Hip Flexors

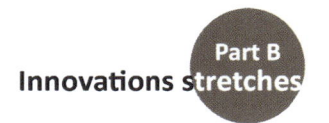

Part B Innovations stretches

HOW TO STRETCH: Photo A
- Kneel next to box, front foot in front of knee
- Keep spine vertical and tilt pelvis backwards
- Tighten abdominal muscles
- Lean hips forwards towards floor

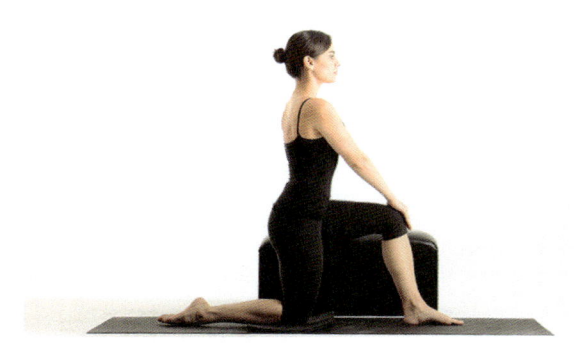

A

HOW TO CONTRACT: Photo B
- Press back knee into floor as if trying to swing the leg forward

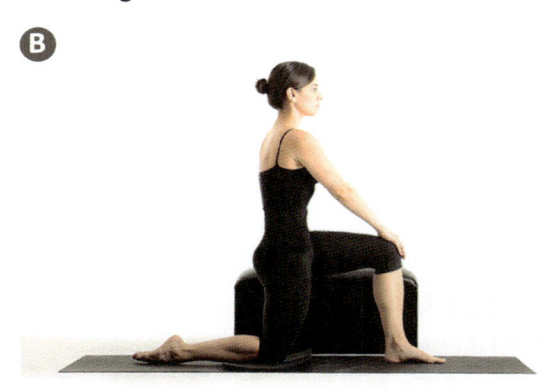

B

HOW TO RESTRETCH: Photo C
- Tuck pelvis further and tighten abdominal muscles
- Press arm down into opposite knee
- Lean hips forwards towards front foot

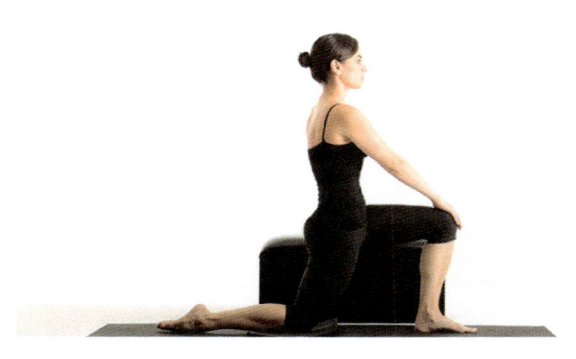

C

PARTNER VARIATION: Photo D
- Partner aligns pelvis horizontally
- Partner presses pelvis towards front foot

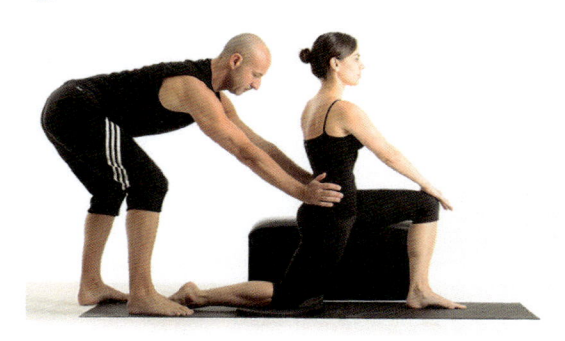

D

Major muscles stretched
- Iliopsoas
  Pectineus
  TFL

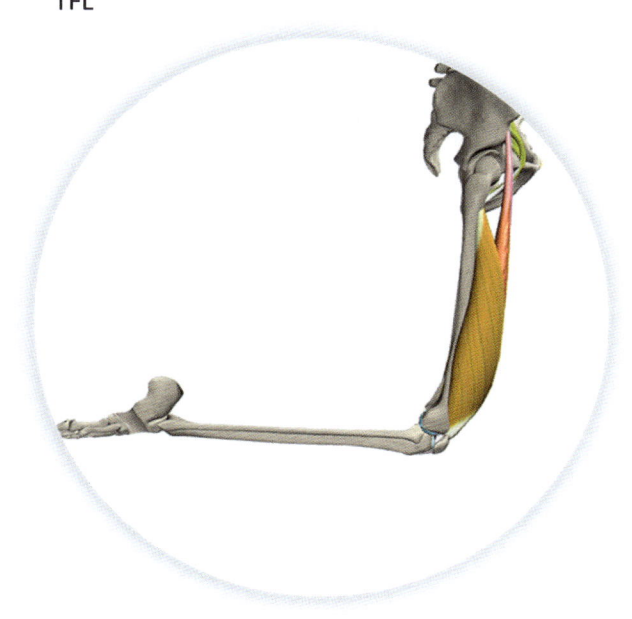

23 Lying Quadricep

Part B
Innovations stretches

HOW TO STRETCH: Photo A
- Lie as pictured, place strap across foot
- Tighten abdominal muscles and press pubic bone into floor
- Pull foot towards bottom

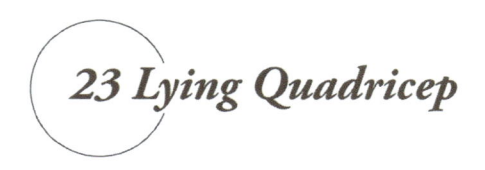

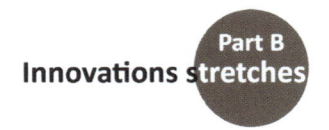

HOW TO CONTRACT: Photo A
- Press foot away from bottom

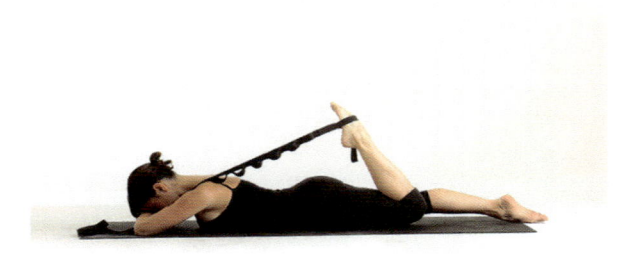

A

HOW TO RESTRETCH: Photo B
- Tighten abdominal muscles again
- Pull foot towards bottom

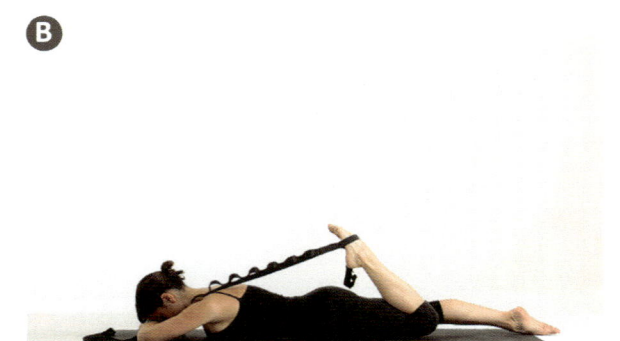

B

Major muscles stretched
- Rectus femoris
- Quadriceps

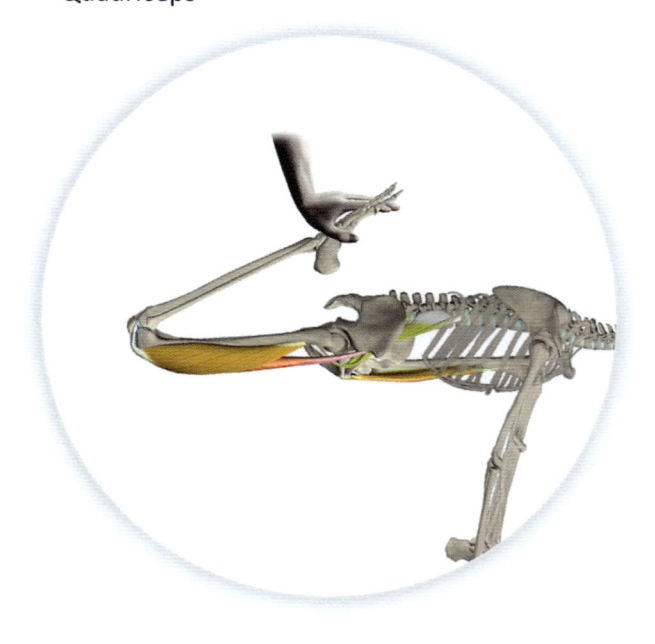

23 Lying Quadricep Variation

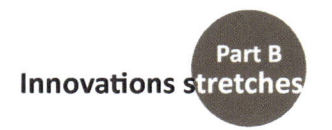

**Part B
Innovations stretches**

Photo C
- Partner takes foot towards bottom
- Partner takes toes towards bottom

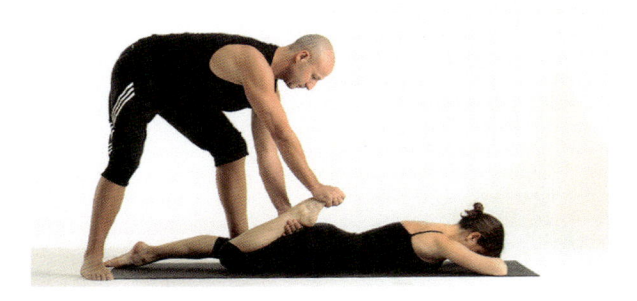

Photo D
- Partner lifts thigh
- Partner keeps heel on bottom

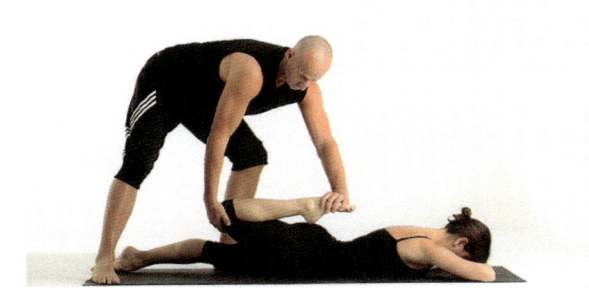

Photo E
- Partner takes thigh away from midline (abduction)

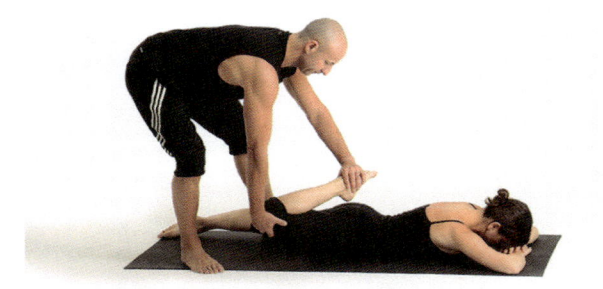

Photo F
- Partner takes thigh towards midline of body to emphasise lateral quad

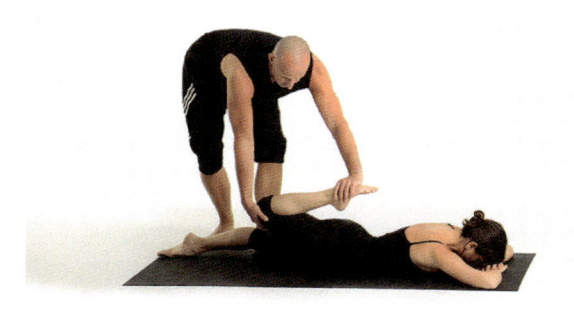

Major muscles stretched
- Rectus femoris
- Iliopsoas
- Quadriceps
  Tibialis anterior

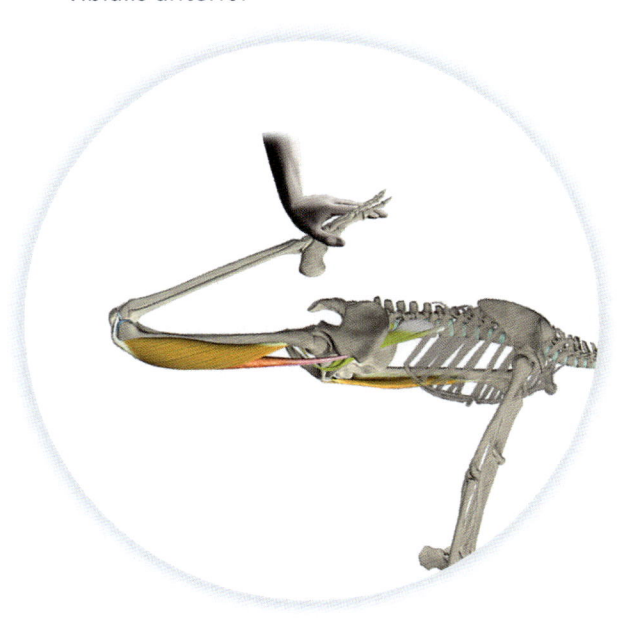

24 Standing Quadricep

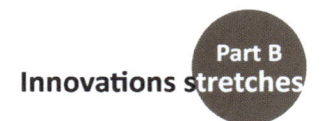

Part B
Innovations stretches

HOW TO STRETCH: Photo A
- Stand as pictured and tighten abdominal muscles to prevent lower back arch (extension)
- Lean bottom back towards foot

HOW TO CONTRACT: Photo A
- Press foot back into box

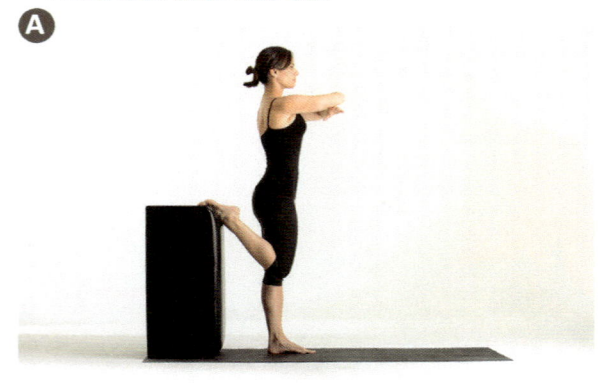

HOW TO RESTRETCH: Photo B
- Tighten abdominal muscles
- Lean bottom back towards foot
- Keep legs parallel

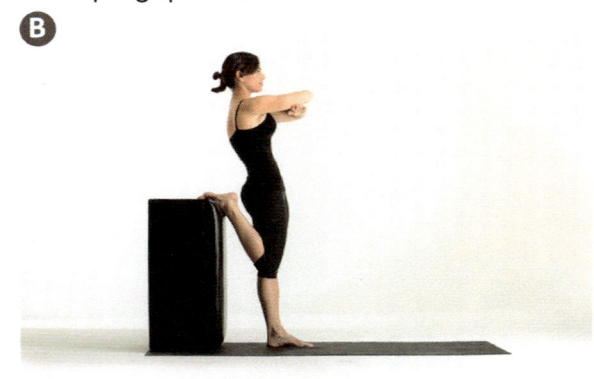

PARTNER: Photo C
- Partner pulls thigh towards box and towards midline of body (adduction)
- Stretchee lifts arm and leans torso towards partner

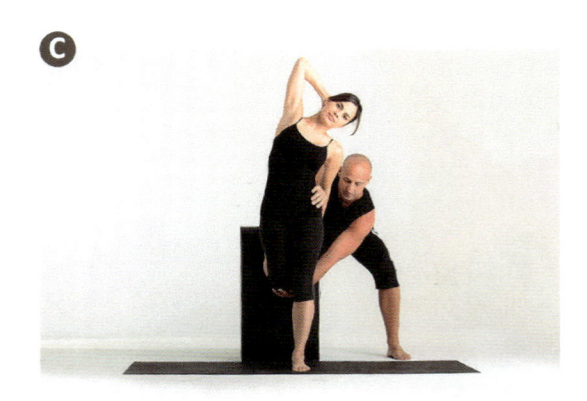

PARTNER: Photo D
- Partner pulls thigh back towards box and away from midline of body

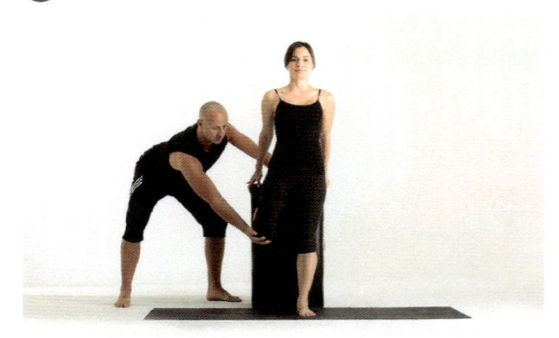

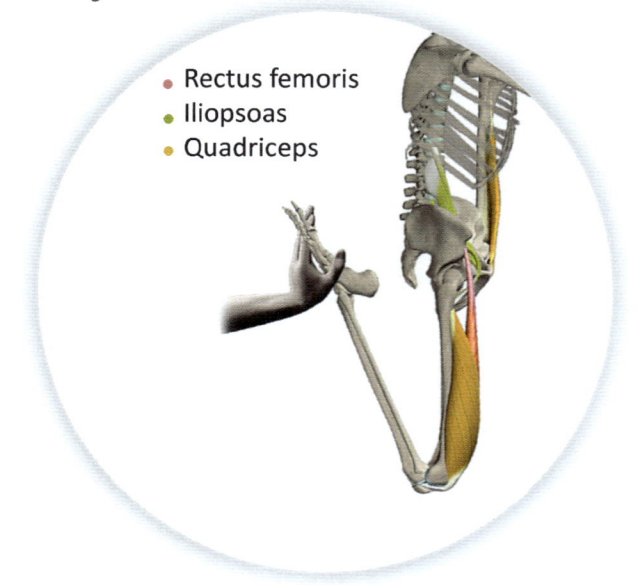

Major muscles stretched

- Rectus femoris
- Iliopsoas
- Quadriceps

25 Floor Godzilla

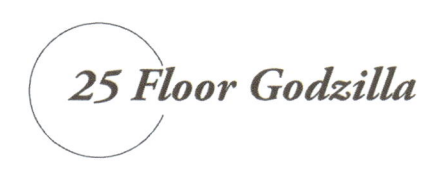

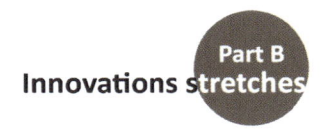

Part B — Innovations stretches

HOW TO STRETCH: Photo A
- Take position as pictured, keeping pelvis neutral
- Pull foot towards bottom
- Keep hips square to line of legs

HOW TO CONTRACT: Photo A
- Press foot away from bottom

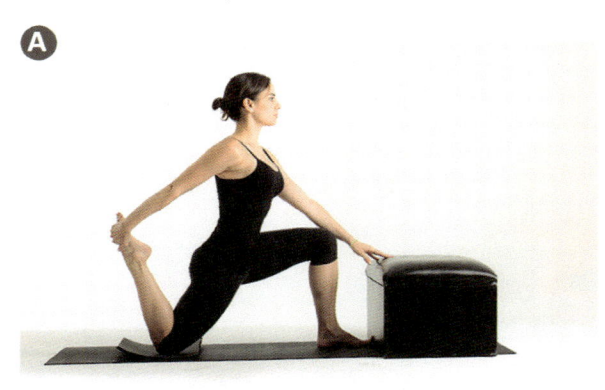

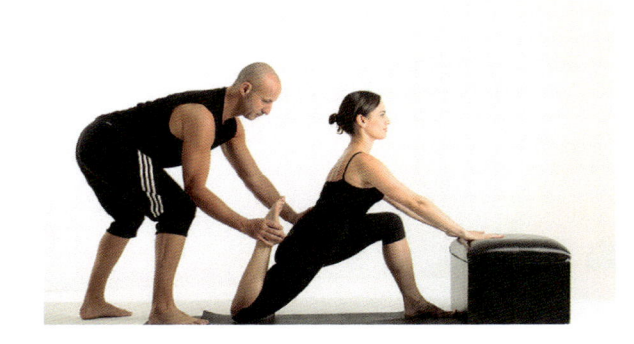

HOW TO RESTRETCH: Photo B
- Pull foot towards bottom
- Lean hips towards floor
- Keep spine vertical and pelvis neutral

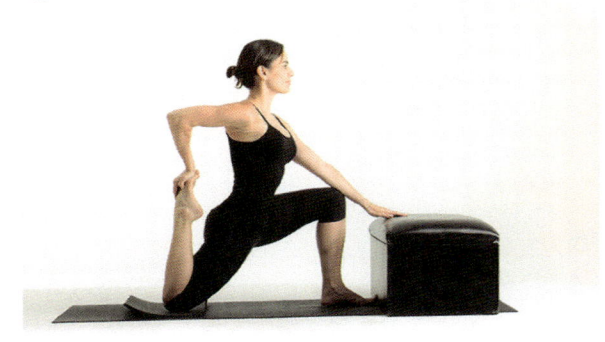

PARTNER VARIATION: Photo C
- Partner presses heel towards bottom and hips towards floor
- Partner keeps hips square

Major muscles stretched
- Rectus femoris
- Iliopsoas
- Quadriceps

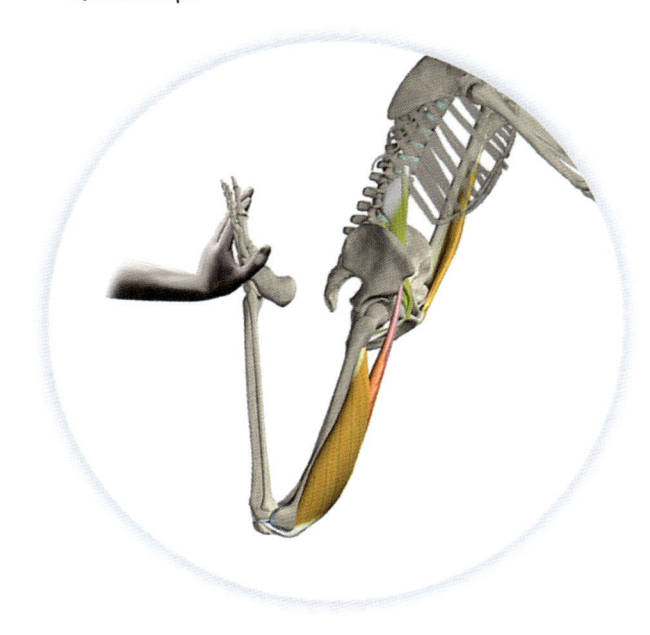

26 Lunge Pose

Part B
Innovations stretches

HOW TO STRETCH: Photo A
- Kneel as pictured, keeping arms inside of front foot
- Keep spine straight
- Take rear leg back as far as possible
- Keep front knee open at about 100° angle
- Sink hips towards floor

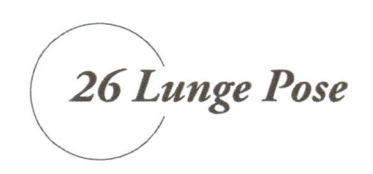

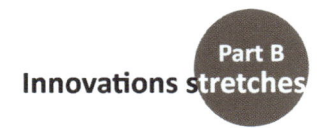

HOW TO CONTRACT: Photo A
- Press both feet down into floor (do not move)

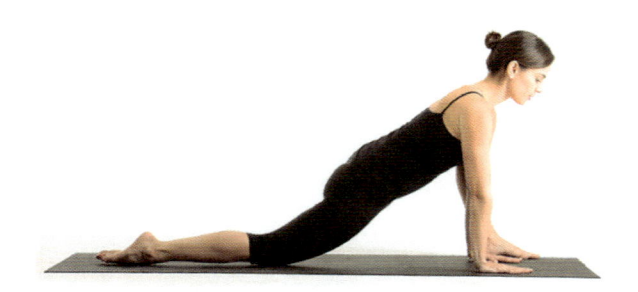

A

HOW TO RESTRETCH: Photo B
- Lean hips closer to floor, OR for more effect lift rear knee from floor (do not allow hips to lift)

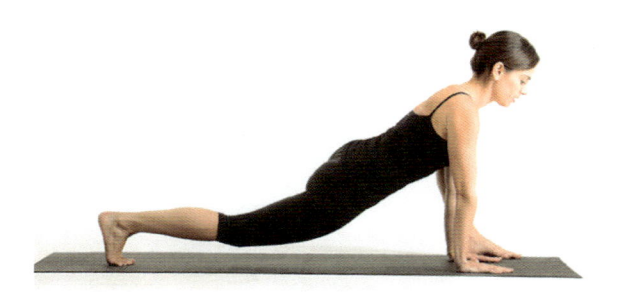

B

PARTNER ASSIST: Photo C
- Partner presses down onto sacrum and rear of hip joint
- Partner lifts leg by pulling thigh up into straight leg position

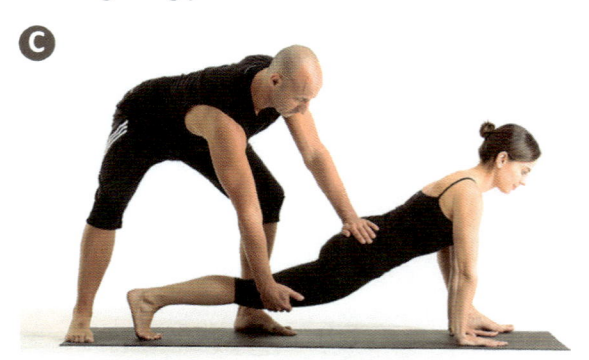

C

Major muscles stretched
- Rectus femoris
- Iliopsoas
- Adductors magnus
- Gluteus maximus

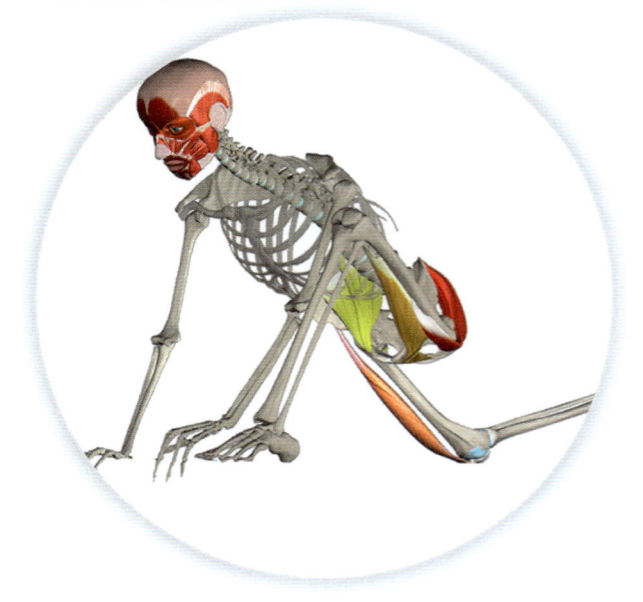

26 Lunge Pose Variation

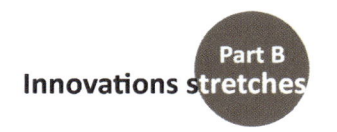

Part B — Innovations stretches

HOW TO STRETCH: Photo D
- Lower yourself onto elbows
- Keep spine straight as possible

HOW TO CONTRACT: Photo D
- Press rear foot into floor

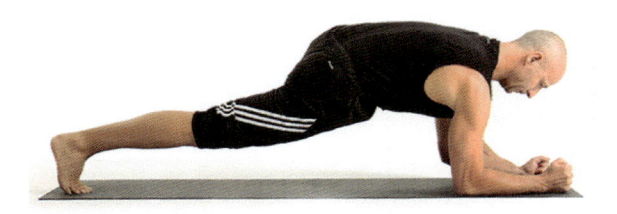

D

HOW TO RESTRETCH: Photo E
- Keep rear leg straight
- Twist spine and pelvis away from rear leg, towards front leg
- Keep hips low to floor

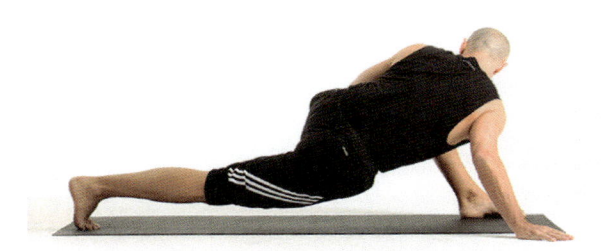

E

Major muscles stretched
- TFL
- Anterior portion of gluteus minimus and medius
- Iliopsoas

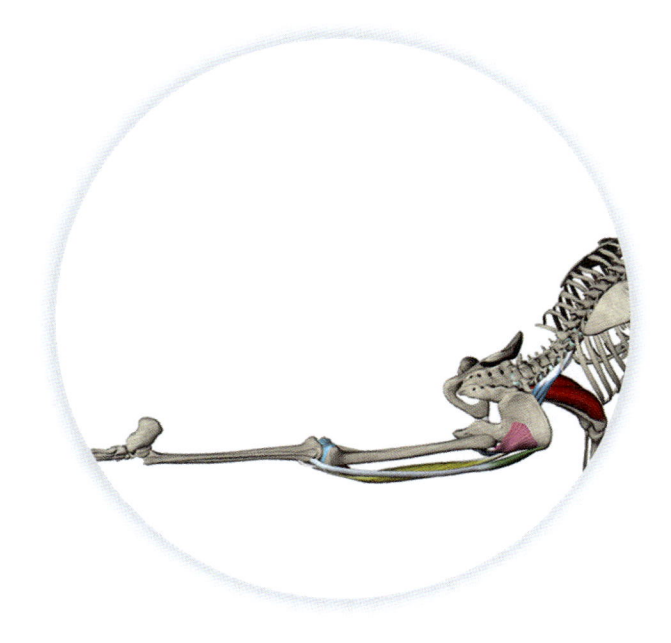

The Gluteal Region
Chapter 4

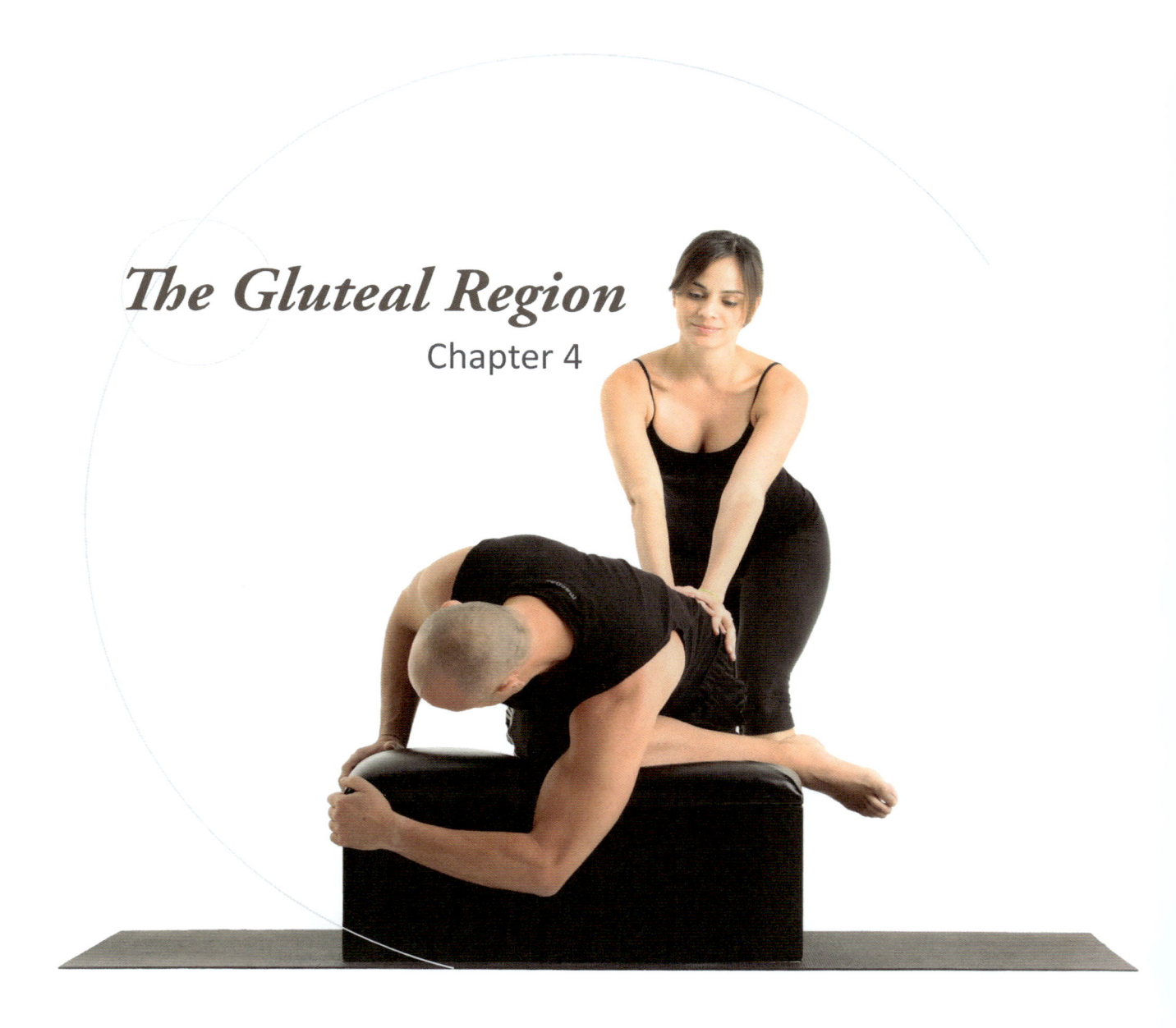

Chapter 4 – Muscle Chart

Hip

Muscle	Flexion	Extension	Adduction	Abduction	Internal rotation	External rotation
Gluteus maximus		●				●
Gluteus medius	●	●		●	●	●
Gluteus minumus	●	●		●	●	●
Tensor fascia lata	●			●	●	
Psoas major	●					●
Iliacus	●					●
Rectus femoris	●			●		
Sartorius	●			●		●
Pectineus	●		●			●
Adductor magnus		●	●			●
Adductor longus	●		●			●
Adductor brevis	●		●			●
Gracilis	●		●			●
Piriformis				●		●
Gemellus superior				●		●
Gemellus inferior				●		●
Obturator internus				●		●
Obturator externus						●
Quadratus femoris			●		●	●
Semitendinosus		●			●	
Semimembranosus		●				
Biceps femoris		●				●

27 Seated Hip

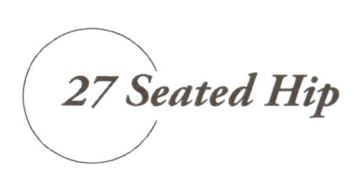

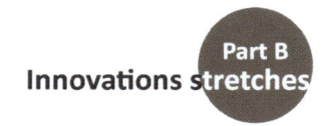

Part B
Innovations stretches

HOW TO STRETCH: Photo A and B
- Hook elbow around opposite knee
- Lift chest
- Keep sit bones on box

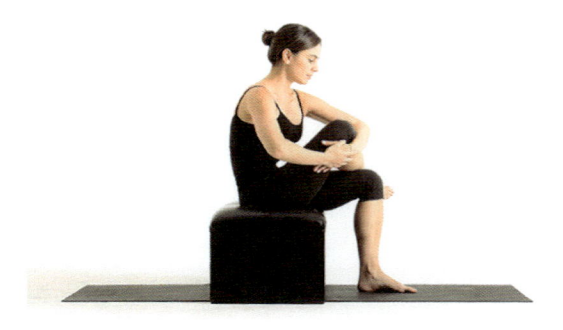

A

HOW TO CONTRACT: Photo B
- Press knee away from armpit

HOW TO RESTRETCH: Photo B
- Pull the knee further to the armpit
- Arch spine
- Twist spine towards the stretching hip

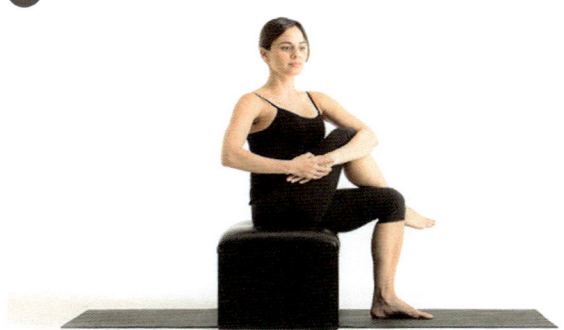

B

Major muscles stretched
Gluteals
Deep rotators

28 Criss Cross

Part B
Innovations stretches

HOW TO STRETCH: Photo A
- Cross leg above knee
- Press leg towards chest
- Keep tailbone on the mat
- Press ankles towards shoulders

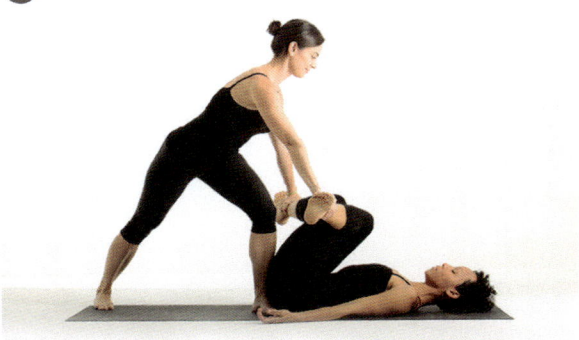

A

HOW TO CONTRACT: Photo B
- Press leg closest to chest away from chest

HOW TO RESTRETCH: Photo B
- Press leg closer to chest
- Press ankles to shoulders

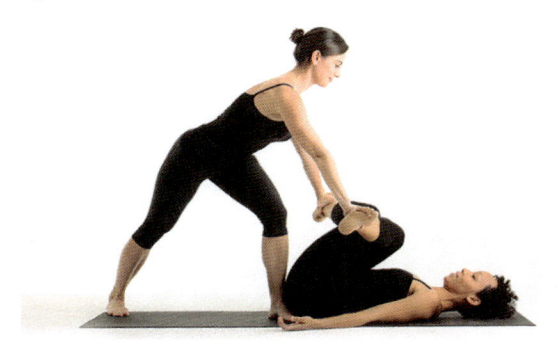

B

Major muscles stretched
- Gluteals
- Deep hip rotators

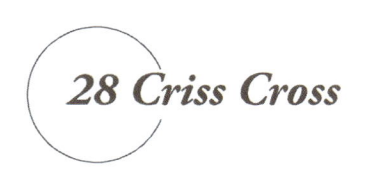

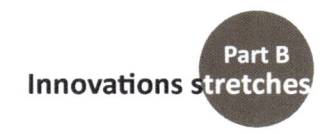

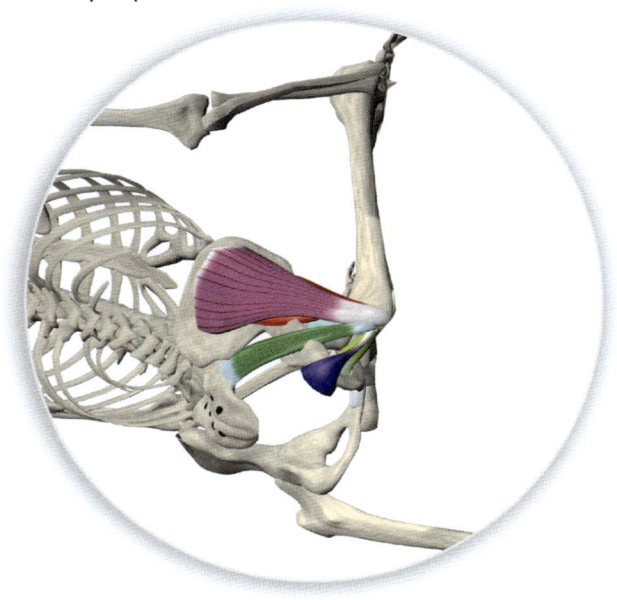

29 Box Pigeon

Part B — Innovations stretches

HOW TO STRETCH: Photo A
- Sit on the box, thigh at 90° to pelvis
- Knee flexed to 90°

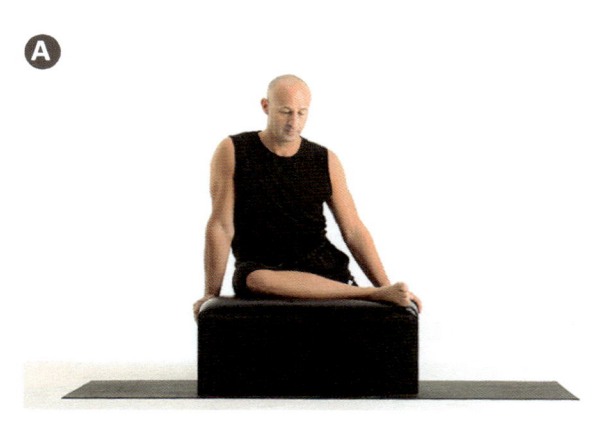

A

HOW TO CONTRACT: Photo B
- Try to level hips
- Press foot on box down towards box

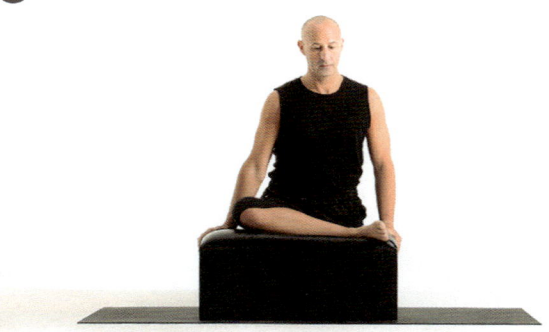

B

HOW TO RESTRETCH: Photo C
- Lean chest towards foot
- Keep spine straight

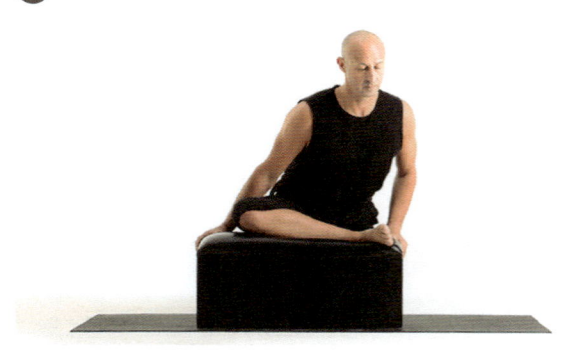

C

PARTNER ASSISTANCE: Photo C
- Partner to press on pelvis to square hips

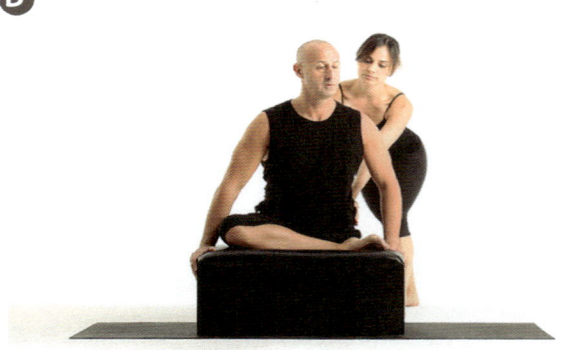

D

Major muscles stretched
- Gluteals
- Deep hip rotators

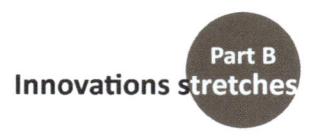

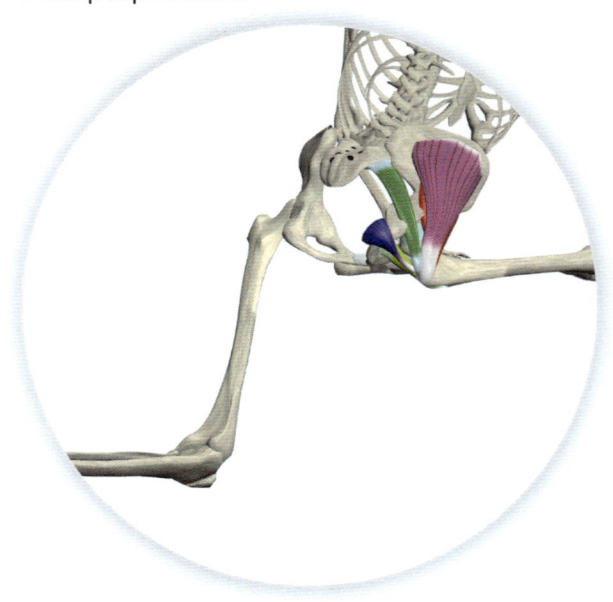

30 Box Twist

**Part B
Innovations stretches**

HOW TO STRETCH: Photo A
- Sit on the box
- Align knee with navel
- Rotate opposite hip towards box

HOW TO CONTRACT: Photo A
- Press front leg into the box to contract
- Square hips to line of leg

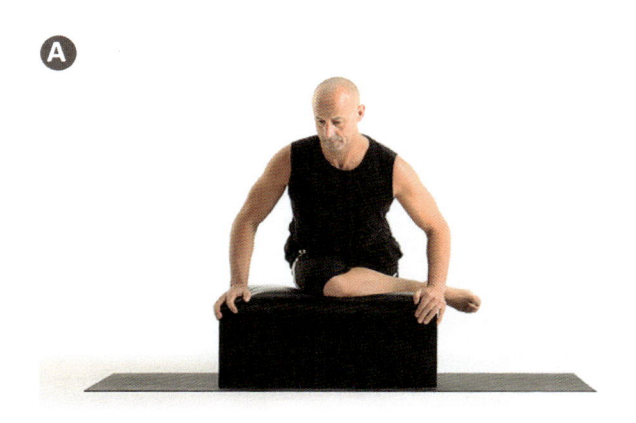

A

HOW TO RESTRETCH: Photo B
- Lower opposite armpit to front knee

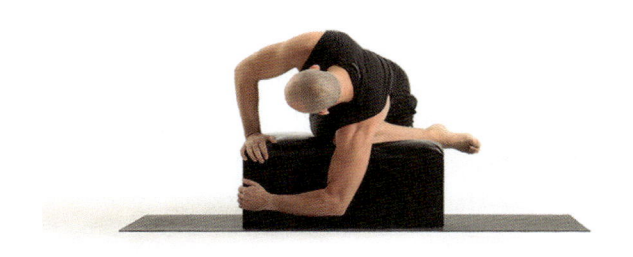

B

PARTNER ASSISTANCE: Photo C
- Partner presses on pelvis to assist with pelvic rotation

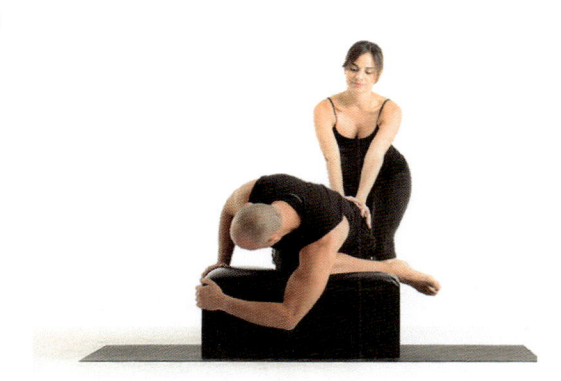

C

Major muscles stretched
- Gluteals
- Deep hip rotators

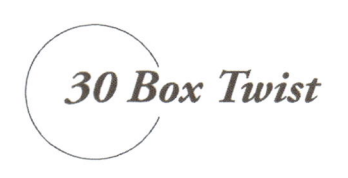

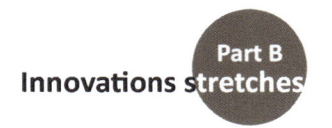

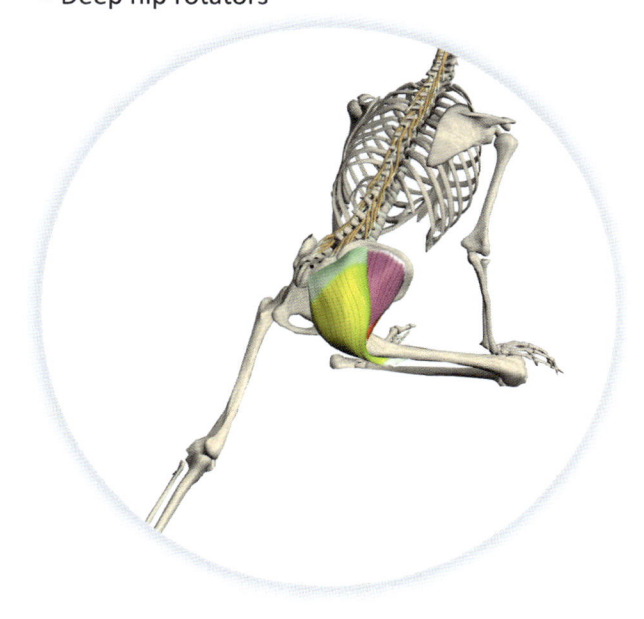

31 Pigeon

Part B
Innovations stretches

HOW TO STRETCH: Photo A
- Sit on the floor, hips square to line of leg
- Front knee at 90°
- Straighten rear leg
- Sit bone of front leg in contact with floor

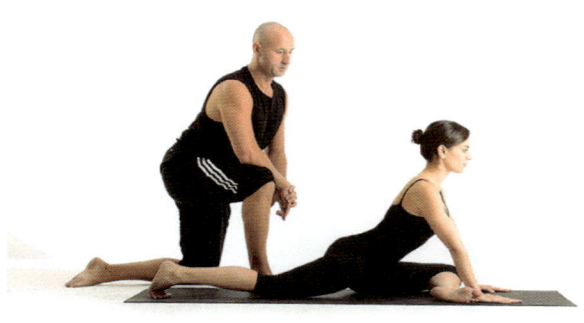

A

HOW TO CONTRACT: Photo B
- Press front foot down into floor

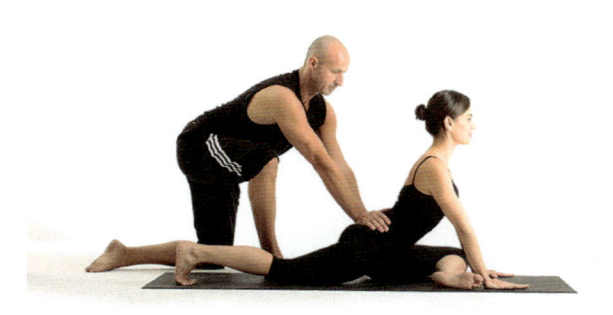

B

HOW TO RESTRETCH: Photo C
- Lean centre of chest towards foot
- Partner to press on pelvis to keep hips square

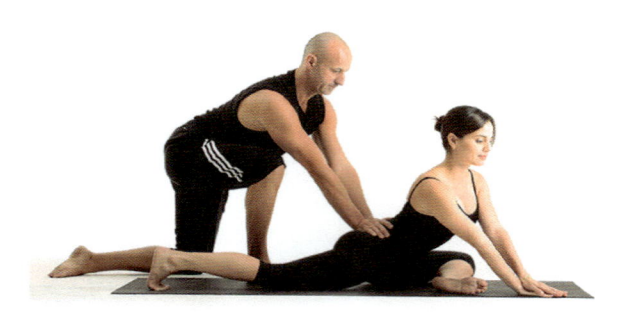

C

Major muscles stretched
- Gluteals
- Deep hip rotators

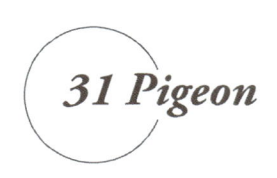

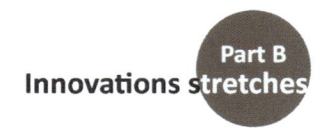

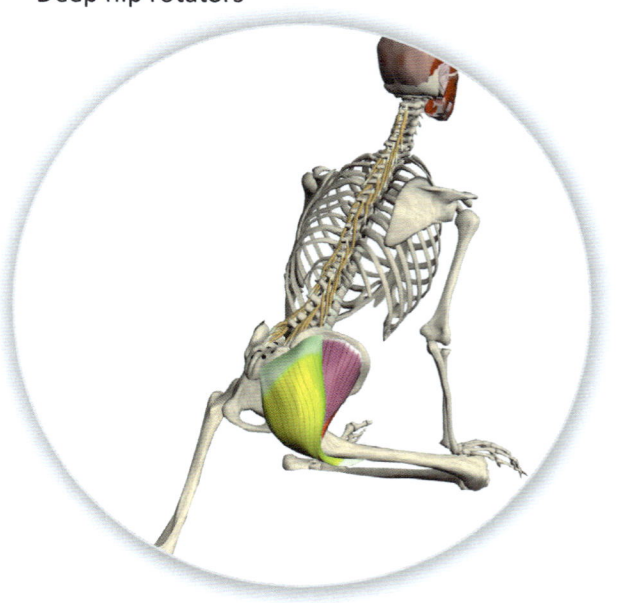

The Adductors
Chapter 5

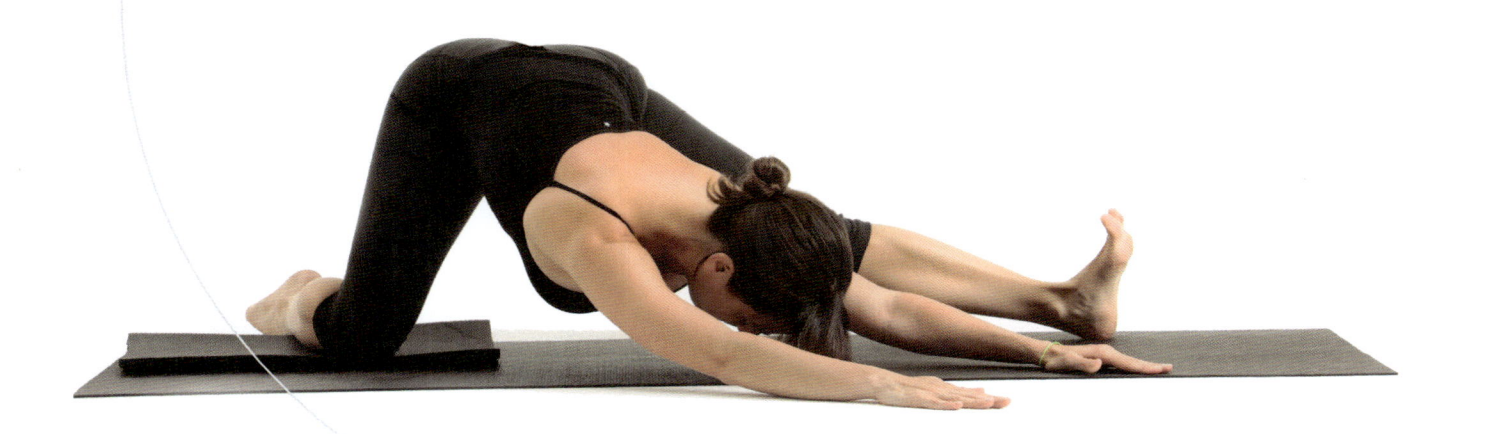

Chapter 5 – Muscle Chart

Hip

Muscle	Flexion	Extension	Adduction	Abduction	Internal rotation	External rotation
Gluteus maximus		●				●
Gluteus medius	●	●		●	●	●
Gluteus minumus	●	●		●	●	●
Tensor fascia lata	●			●	●	
Psoas major	●					●
Iliacus	●					●
Rectus femoris	●			●		
Sartorius	●			●		●
Pectineus	●		●			
Adductor magnus		●	●			●
Adductor longus	●		●			●
Adductor brevis	●		●			●
Gracilis	●		●			
Piriformis				●		●
Gemellus superior				●		●
Gemellus inferior				●		●
Obturator internus				●		●
Obturator externus						●
Quadratus femoris			●		●	●
Semitendinosus		●			●	
Semimembranosus		●				
Biceps femoris		●				●

Knee

Muscle	Flexion	Extension	Internal rotation	External rotation
Vastus medialis		●		
Vastus lateralis		●		
Vastus intermedius		●		
Rectus femoris		●		
Sartorius	●			●
Semitendinosus	●		●	
Semimembranosus	●		●	
Biceps femoris	●			●
Gracilis	●		●	
Popliteus	●			
Gastrocnemius	●			

32 The Frog

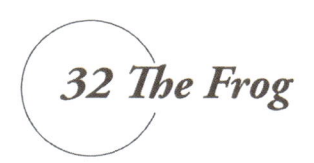

Part B — Innovations stretches

HOW TO STRETCH: Photo A
- Place knee under hips and slowly take legs apart
- Partner to press lightly onto sacrum

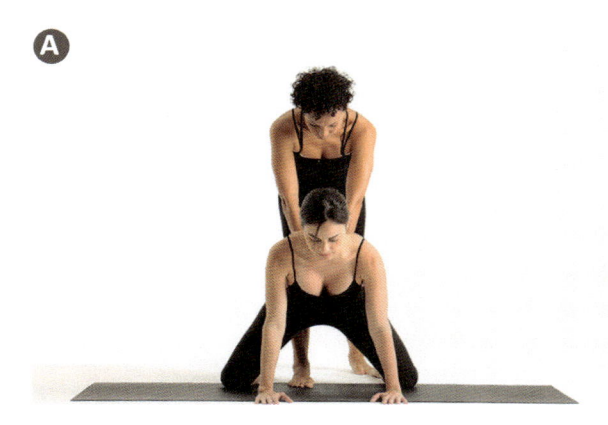

A

HOW TO CONTRACT: Photo B
- Lower yourself onto elbows if you are comfortable
- Press knees towards each other

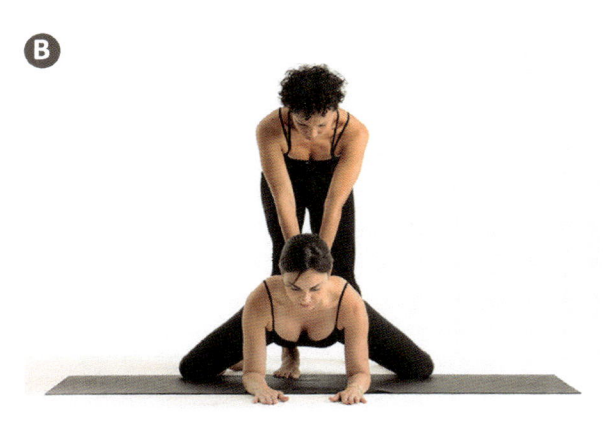

B

HOW TO RESTRETCH: Photo C
- Slide knees further apart
- Partner to lean more weight
- Twist to one side and the other (Photo D)
- Lean hips back and forth to vary the stretch

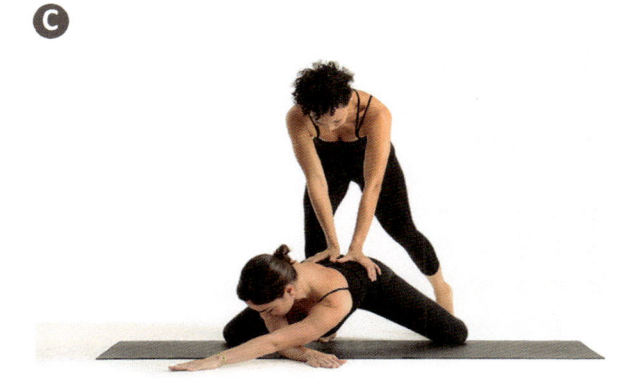

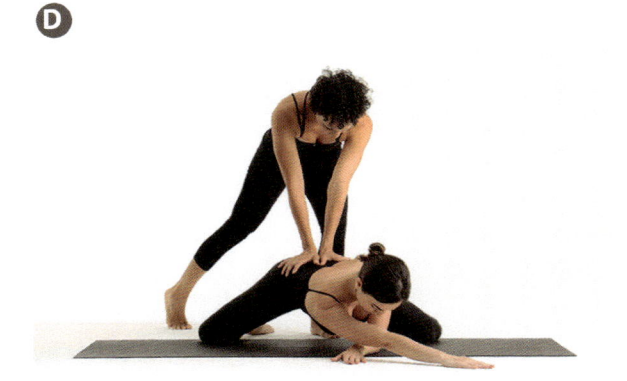

C

D

Major muscles stretched
- Gracilis
- Pectineus
- Adductors brevis
- Adductors longus

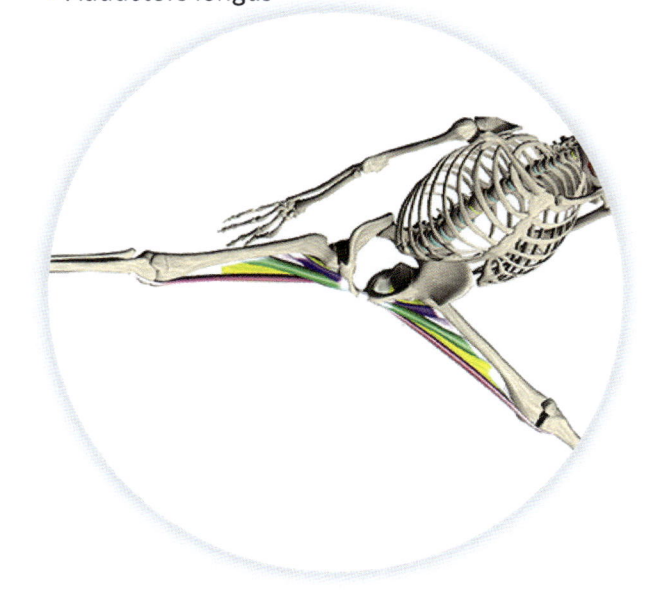

33 Kneeling Short Long

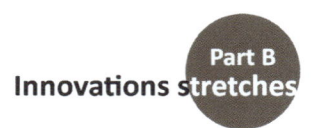

Part B
Innovations stretches

HOW TO STRETCH: Photo A
- Place even weight on hands and legs
- Lean to one side at a time
- Lean hips fowards and backwards also

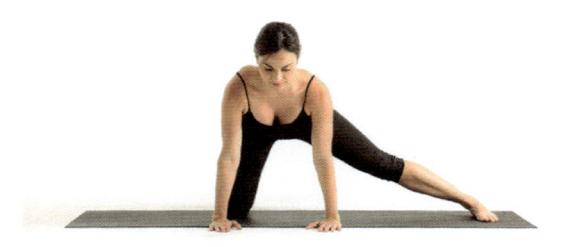

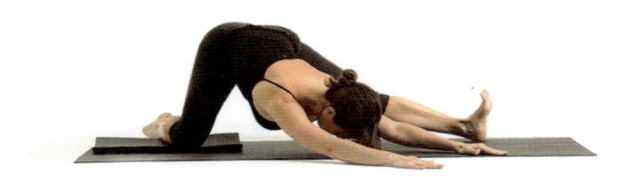

A

HOW TO CONTRACT: Photo B
- Lower yourself onto elbows if possible
- Press knee and foot into the mat

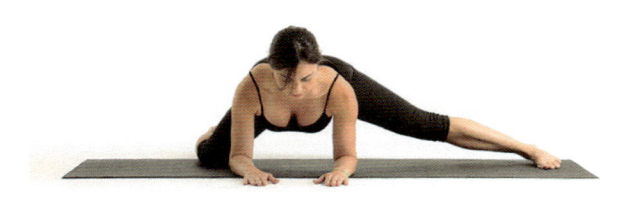

B

HOW TO RESTRETCH: Photo C
- Spread legs further apart
- Twist trunk to both legs (Photos C, D)

C

VARIATION: Photo D
- Externally rotate straight leg for hamstring focus

D

Major muscles stretched
- Gracilis
- Pectineus
- Adductors brevis
- Adductors longus

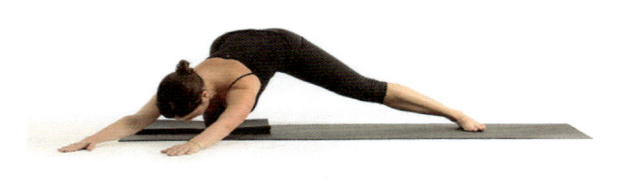

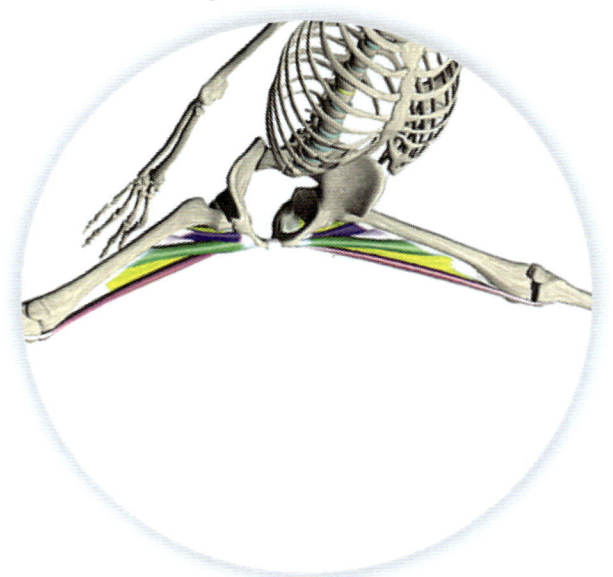

34 Lying Adductors

Part B — Innovations stretches

HOW TO STRETCH: Photo A
- Position bottom and legs against wall
- Slowly take the legs apart
- Pull slightly on straps

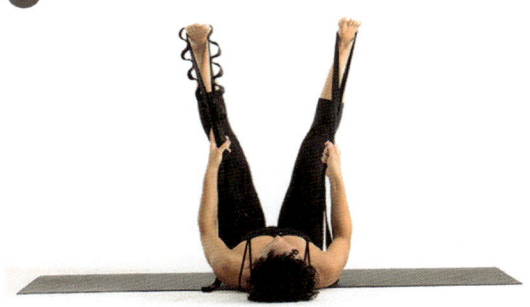

A

HOW TO CONTRACT: Photo B
- Tighten quadriceps
- Press legs to each other
- Prevent movement with strap

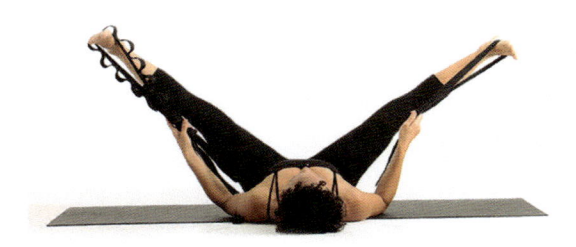

B

Major muscles stretched
- Gracilis
- Pectineus
- Adductors brevis
- Adductors longus

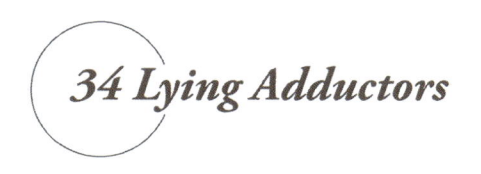

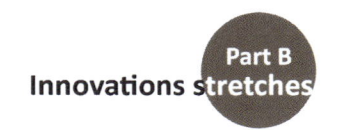

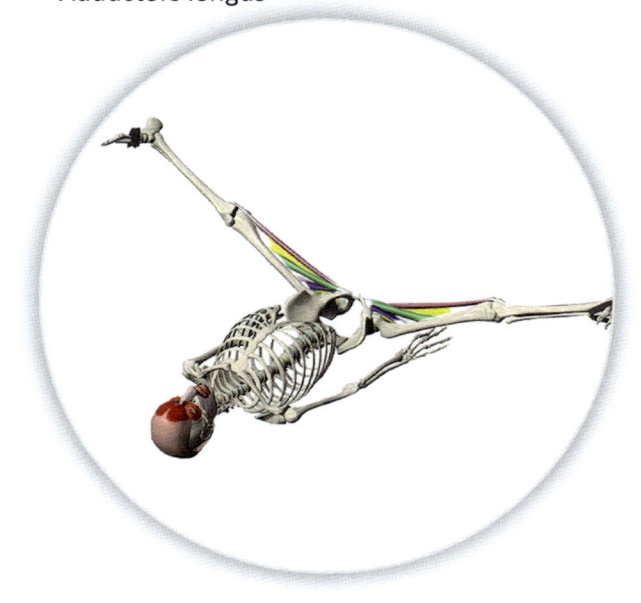

HOW TO RESTRETCH: Photo C
- Gently allow legs apart
- Pull lightly on strap

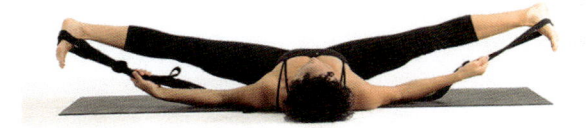

C

35 Seated Partner Adductors

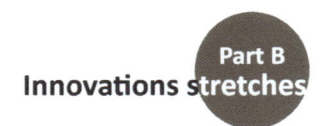

Part B
Innovations stretches

HOW TO STRETCH: Photo A
- Sit against base
- Pelvis neutral
- Feet together
- Partner rests feet gently on thighs

HOW TO CONTRACT: Photo A
- Press thighs up into partner's feet

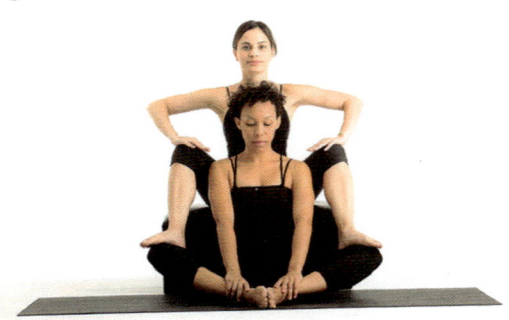

A

HOW TO RESTRETCH: Photo B
- Press down into thighs

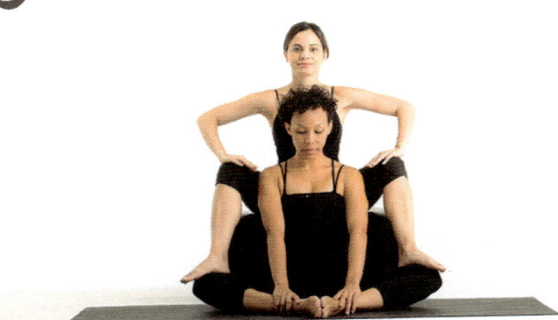

B

ALTERNATIVE POSITION
Identical instructions as above except:
- Partner uses hands instead of feet
- Stretcher lies on foor with neutral spine

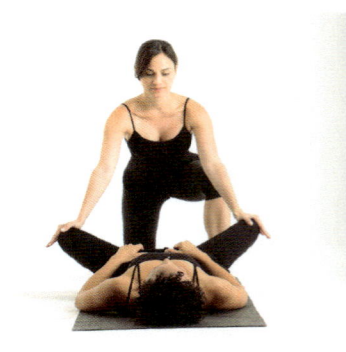

C

Major muscles stretched
- Gracilis
- Pectineus
- Adductors brevis
- Adductors longus

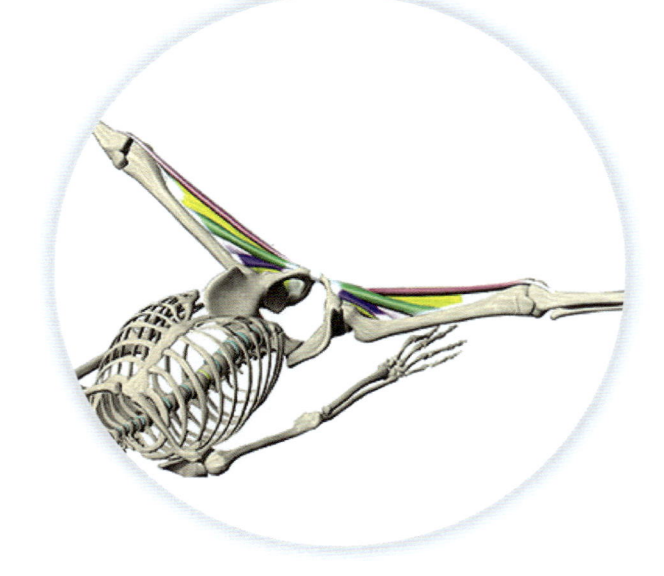

36 Seated Bent Leg Split

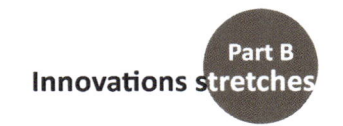

Part B — Innovations stretches

HOW TO STRETCH: Photo A
- Take legs away from centre
- Keep knees bent

HOW TO CONTRACT: Photo A
- Press heels into the floor
- Press thighs into arms towards the centre

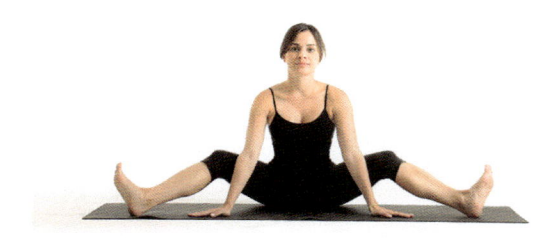

A

HOW TO RESTRETCH: Photo B
- With caution, try to straighten legs
- Keep legs apart
- Allow lower back to extend (not shown)

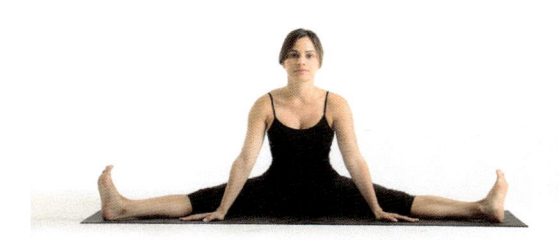

B

Major muscles stretched
- Gracilis
- Pectineus
- Adductors brevis
- Adductors longus

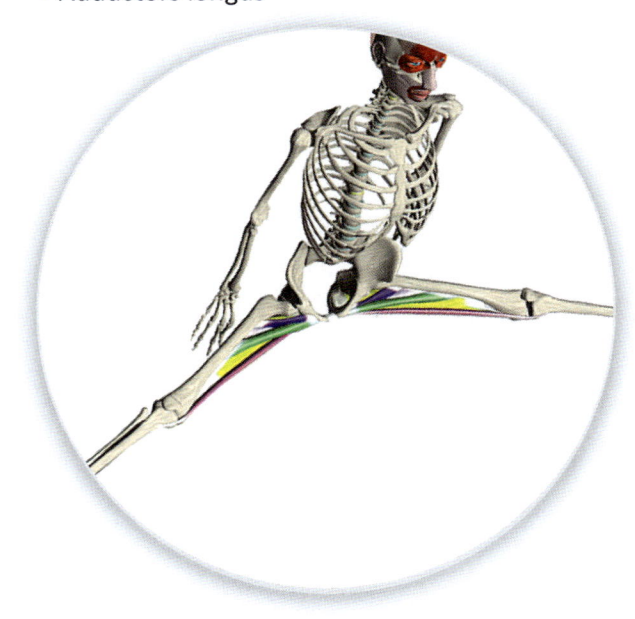

The Trunk
Chapter 6

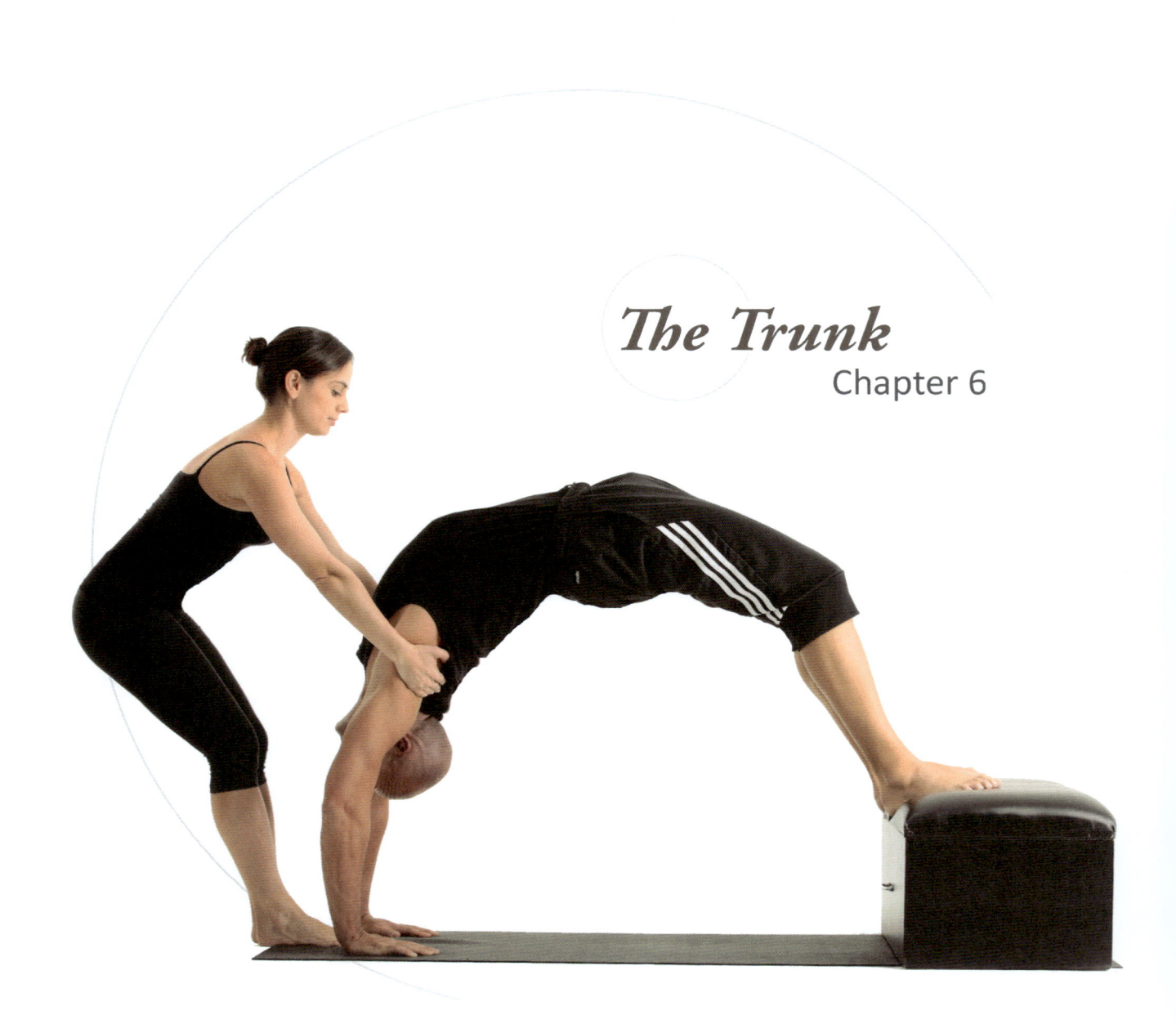

Chapter 6 – Muscle Chart

Trunk

Muscle	Flexion	Extension	Lateral flexion	Rotation
External oblique	●		●	●
Internal oblique	●		●	●
Rectus abdominis	●			
Spinalis thoracis		●		
Lateral intertransversi			●	
Interspinalis		●		
Longissimus thoracis		●		
Iliocostalis lumborum		●		
Multifidus		●		
Rotatores		●		●
Quadratus lumborum		●	●	
Psoas major	●		●	
Iliacus	●		●	

37 The Accelerator

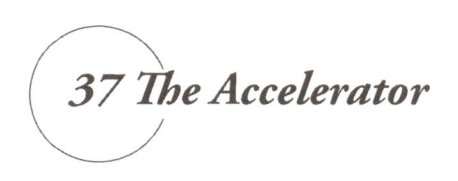

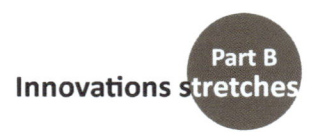

Part B Innovations stretches

FLEXION

HOW TO STRETCH: Photo A
- Clasp wrists around thighs
- Roll pelvis backwards (posterior tilt)
- Allow whole spine to round
- Tighten abdominal muscles

HOW TO CONTRACT: Photo A
- Try to pull shoulder blades together

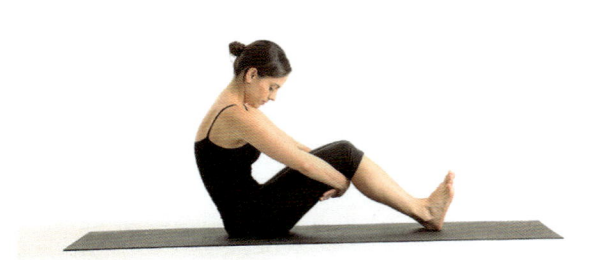

A

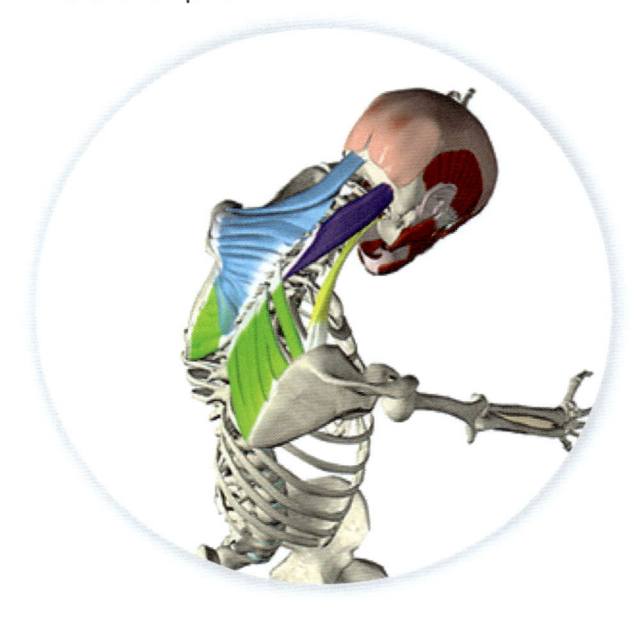

HOW TO RESTRETCH: Photo B
- Slide one heel further away
- Tilt head to opposite shoulder
- Repeat on opposite leg

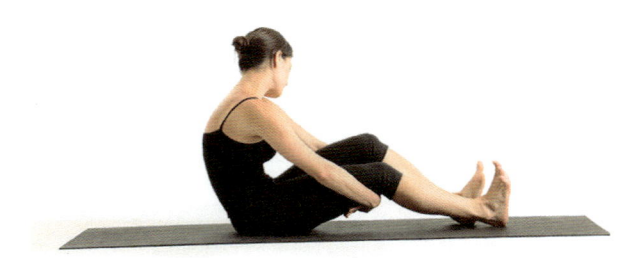

B

Major muscles stretched
- Posterior deltoid
- Middle trapezius
- Rhomboids
- Levator scapula

Major muscles stretched
- Rhomboids
- Middle trapezius

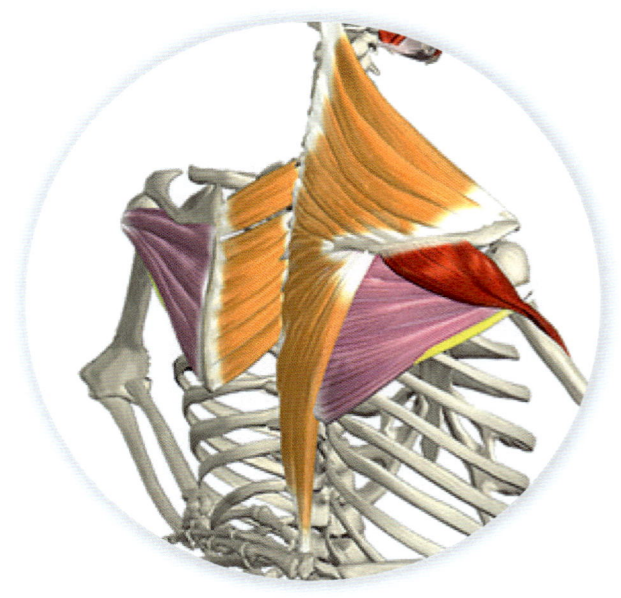

38 The Dangler

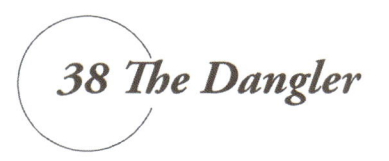

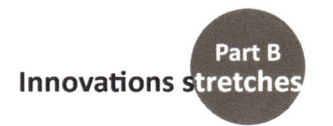

Part B Innovations stretches

FLEXION
HOW TO STRETCH: Photo A
- Lie over box with pubic bone off the edge
- Allow head and knees to drop completely
- Take deep abdominal breaths

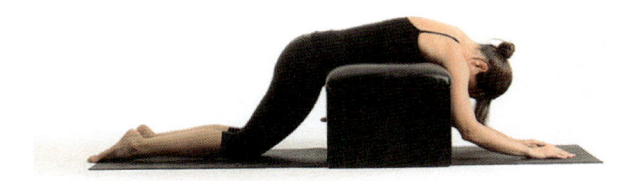

A

HOW TO CONTRACT: Photo B
- Imagine pressing legs and head/upper back to ceiling

HOW TO RESTRETCH: Photo B
- Let hips and head drop down to floor
- Allow legs to float as much as possible

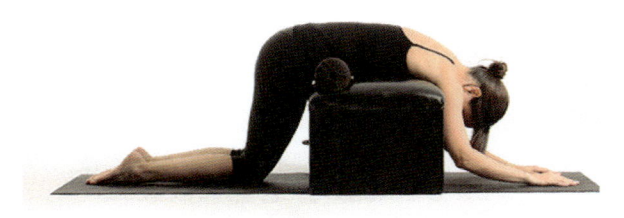

B

Photo C
- Stronger versions with less floor contact
- Instructions as above

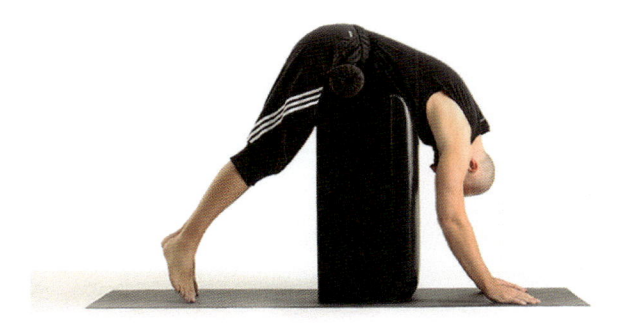

C

PARTNER VARIATION: Photo D
- Allow legs and upper body to dangle
- Contract by pushing pelvis/chest up into partner resistance
- Restretch by hanging further
- Deep abdominal breaths are important

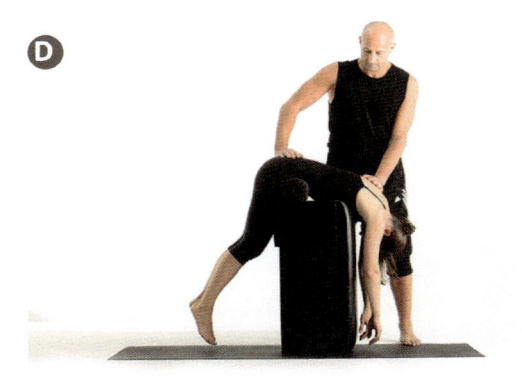

D

Major muscles stretched
- Erector spinae
- Rhomboids

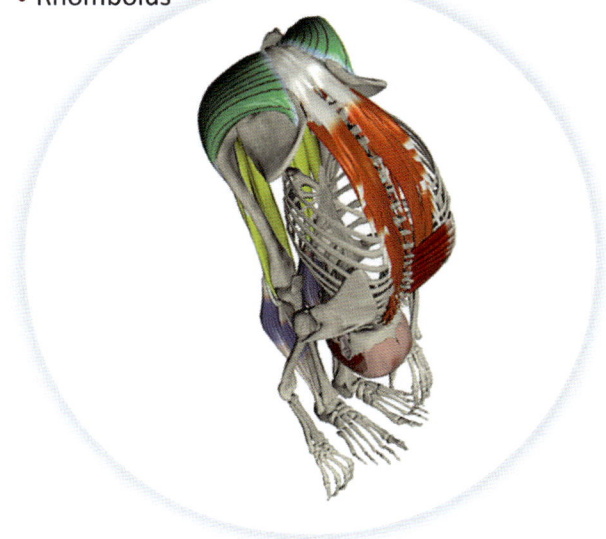

39 The Cat

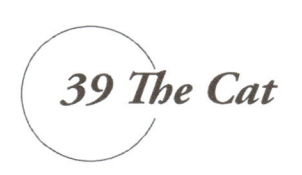

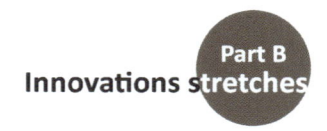

Part B — Innovations stretches

FLEXION

HOW TO SET UP: Photo A
- Find neutral spine
- Support shoulders keeping scapular flat on ribs

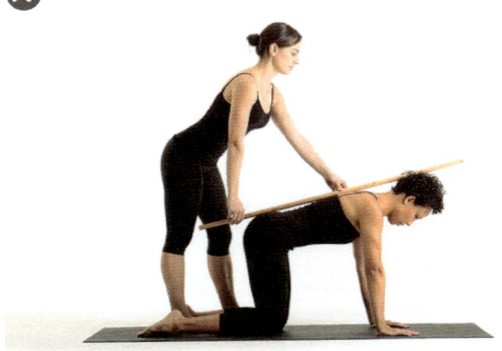

A

HOW TO CONTRACT: Photo B
- Tuck bottom under
- Contract abdominal muscles
- Take chin to chest
- Press hands outwards to stretch between shoulder blades
- Press hands away from knees to stretch upper trapezius muscles

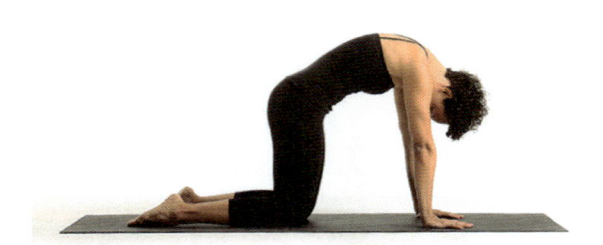

B

Major muscles stretched
- Erector spinae
- Rhomboids

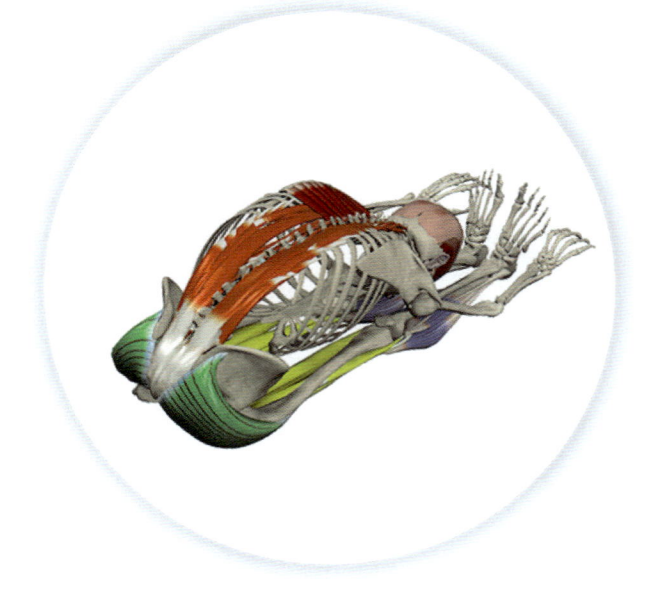

40 Hamstring Spine Combo

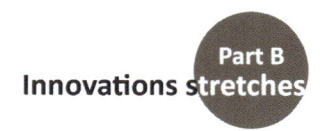

Part B
Innovations stretches

FLEXION

HOW TO STRETCH: Photo A
- Bend one knee and drop it out to the side
- Clasp opposite foot and pull back towards you
- Partner to press on pelvis towards neutral position

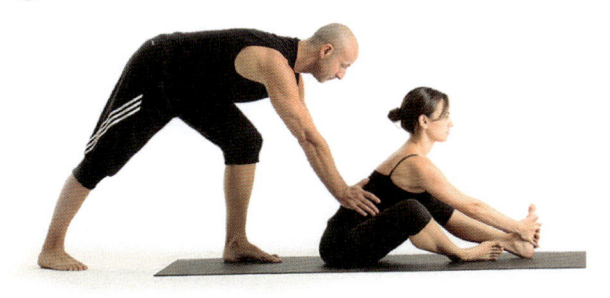

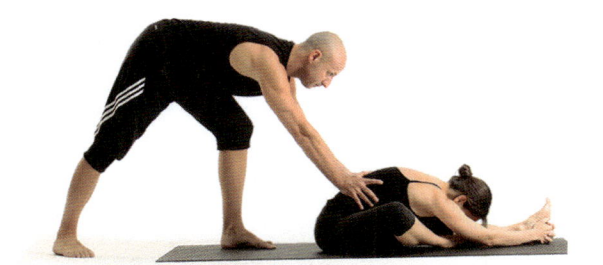

HOW TO CONTRACT: Photo B
- Press heel of foot into floor
- Press ball of foot into hand

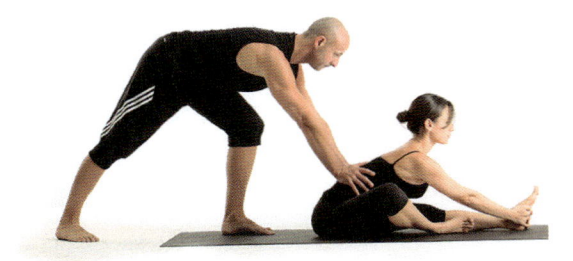

HOW TO RESTRETCH: Photo C
- Straighten leg if possible
- Partner to roll pelvis forwards as much as possible
- Lower chest and head onto leg

Major muscles stretched
- Hamstrings
- Calves
- Erector spinae

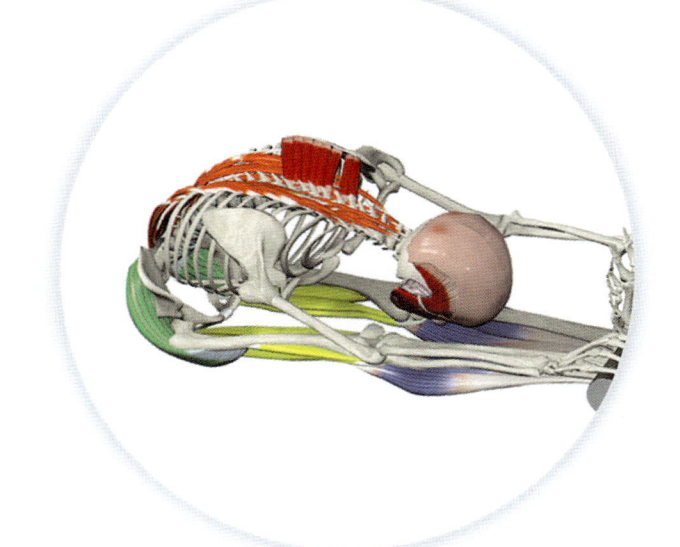

41 BOSU Back Bend

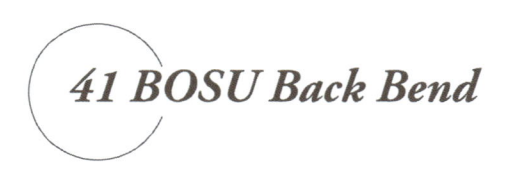

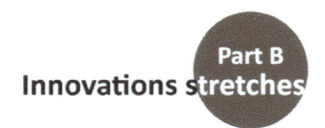

Part B
Innovations stretches

EXTENSION
HOW TO STRETCH: Photo A
- Clasp stick and lie back over BOSU with head supported
- Partner to pull lightly on stick, both backwards and downwards
- Other partner to press lightly onto upper thighs
- Allow pelvis to sink into floor

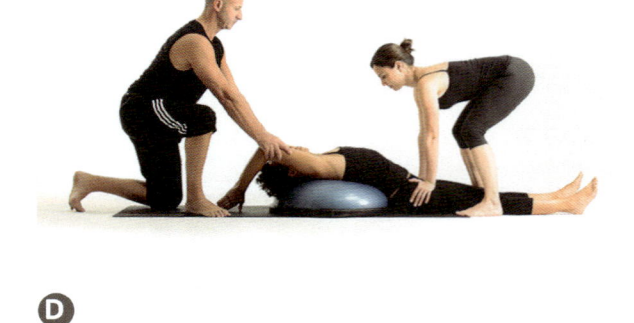

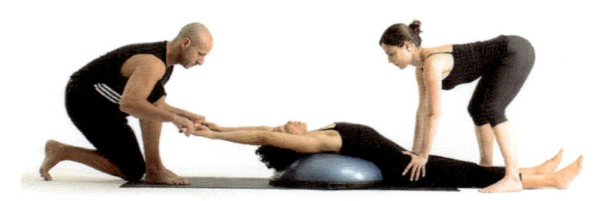

HOW TO CONTRACT: Photo B
- Press arms and thighs towards ceiling for five seconds
- Pull stick towards head for another five seconds

HOW TO RESTRETCH: Photo B
- Allow pelvis to relax into floor
- Pull arms backwards and downwards

ALTERNATIVE ARM POSITION: Photo C
- Clasp hands together and bend elbows
- Pull elbows back and downwards

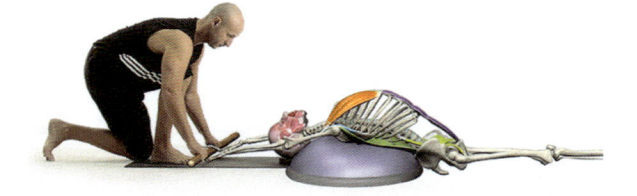

VARIATION: Photo D
- Pull one side of the stick in horizontal plane for lat focus

Major muscles stretched
- Abdominals
- Pectorals
- Latissimus dorsi
- Teres major

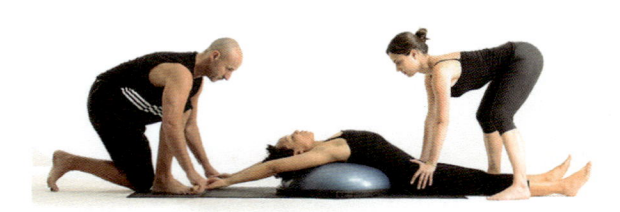

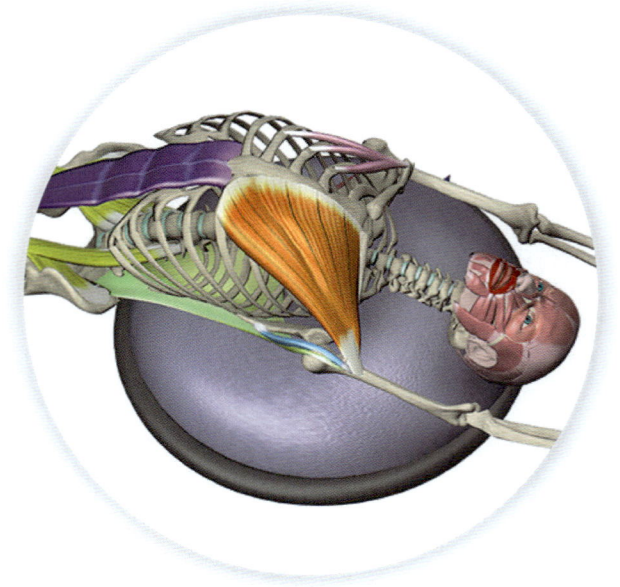

42 The Cobra

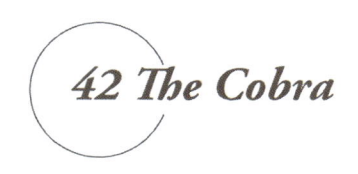

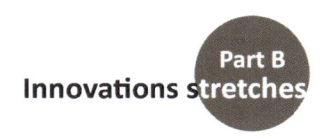

Part B — Innovations stretches

EXTENSION

HOW TO STRETCH: Photo A
- Relax lower back and gluteal muscles
- Draw elbows towards body and lift chest

HOW TO CONTRACT: Photo A
- Press arms and feet into floor

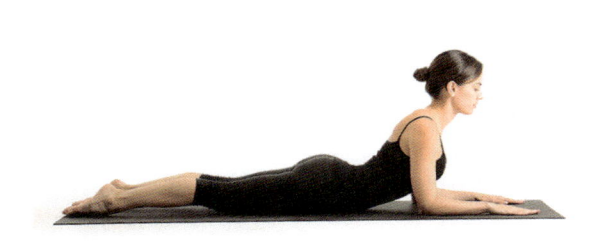

Ⓐ

HOW TO RESTRETCH: Photo B
- Take hands wider than mat
- Relax low back muscles
- Press arms straight to lift chest

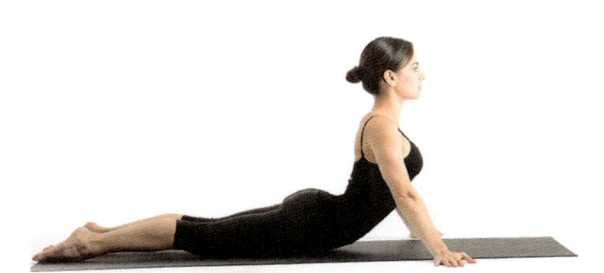

Ⓑ

INTERMEDIATE VARIATION: Photo C
- Lower chest and bring hands closer together onto mat
- Press arms straight and lock elbows
- Relax and 'hang' spine between shoulders
- Deep abdominal breathing

ADVANCED VARIATION: Photo D
- Bring hands closer to hips under shoulders
- Contract leg and spinal muscles to lift knees and hips
- Contract back muscles to arch spine backwards

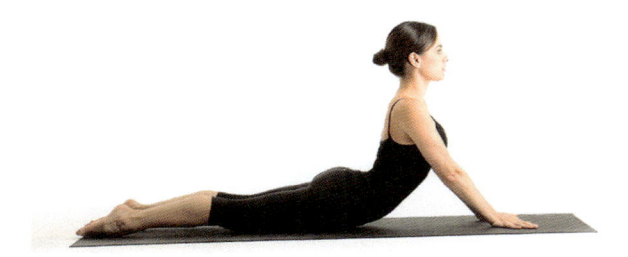

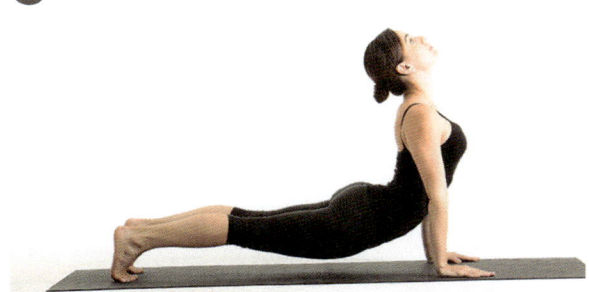

Ⓒ

Ⓓ

Major muscles stretched

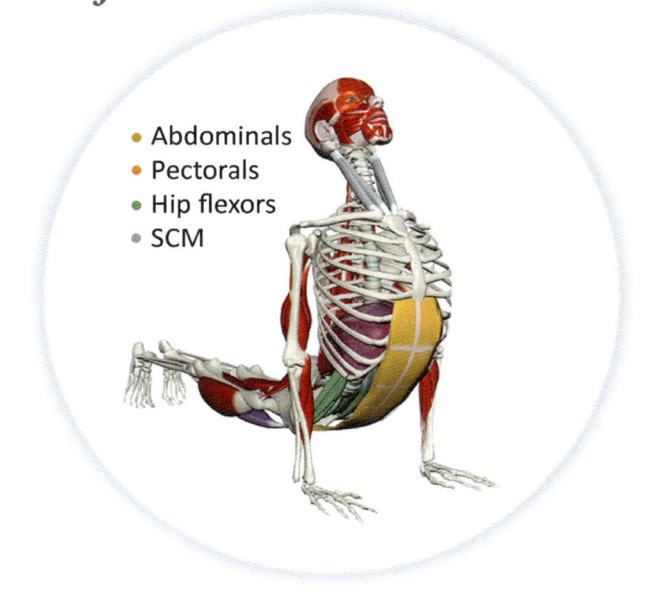

- Abdominals
- Pectorals
- Hip flexors
- SCM

43 Box Wheel

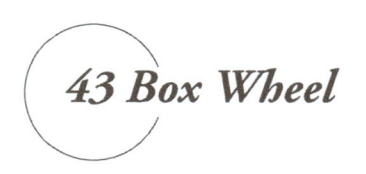

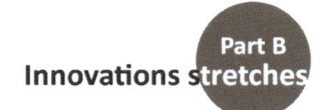

**Part B
Innovations stretches**

EXTENSION

HOW TO SET UP: Photo A
- Place arches of feet onto box, thighs vertical
- Place hands behind shoulders, fingers facing shoulders

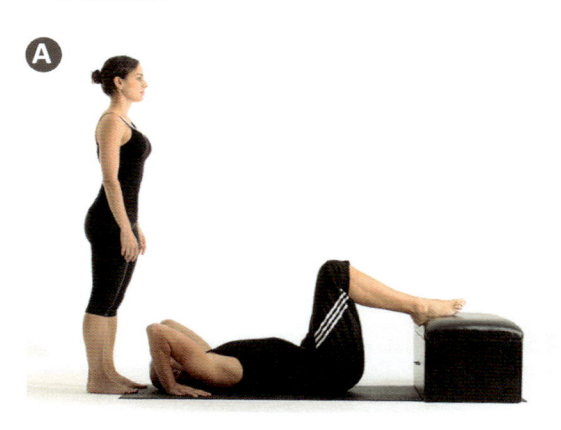

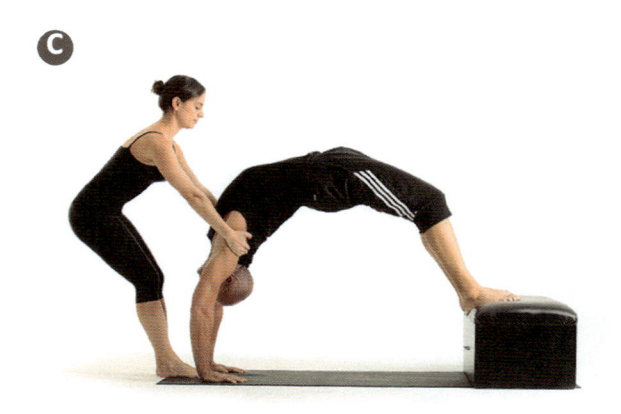

A

HOW TO STRETCH: Photo B
- Press hands and feet towards floor
- Lift body up onto head
- Partner to clasp shoulders

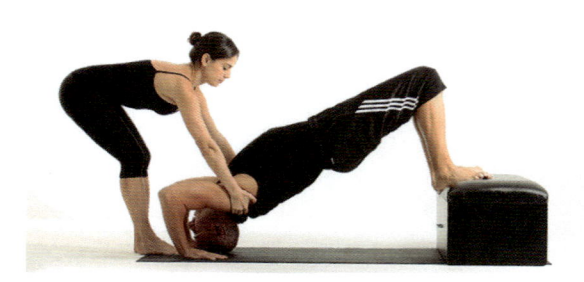

B

HOW TO STRETCH: Photo C
- Press up to final position
- Straighten arms
- Partner to pull chest over the top of hands

C

Major muscles stretched
- Pectorals
- Hip flexors
- Latissimus dorsi
- Abdominals

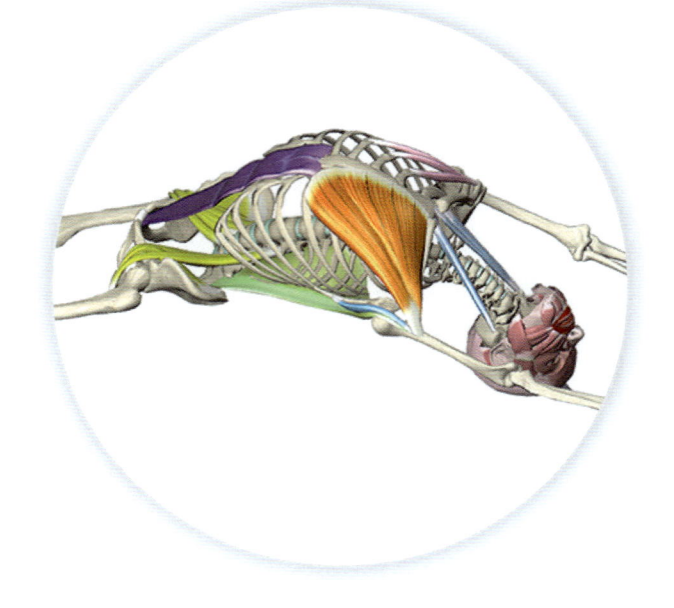

44 Floor Wheel

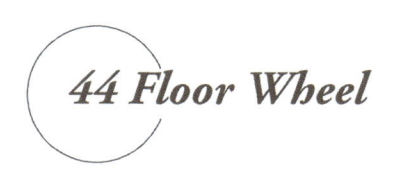

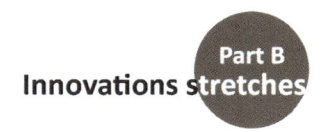

Part B
Innovations stretches

EXTENSION

HOW TO SET UP: Photo A
- Lie on box with sacrum and shoulders just over box edge, fingers facing box

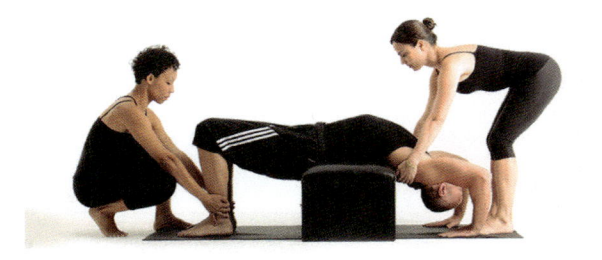

A

HOW TO STRETCH: Photo B
- Push hands and feet into floor to raise chest and hips
- Try to move hands and feet closer together (not pictured)

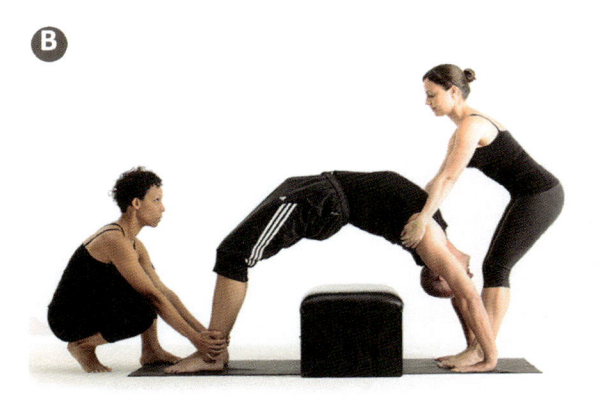

B

Major muscles stretched
- Pectorals
- Hip flexors
- Latissimus dorsi
- Abdominals
- SCM

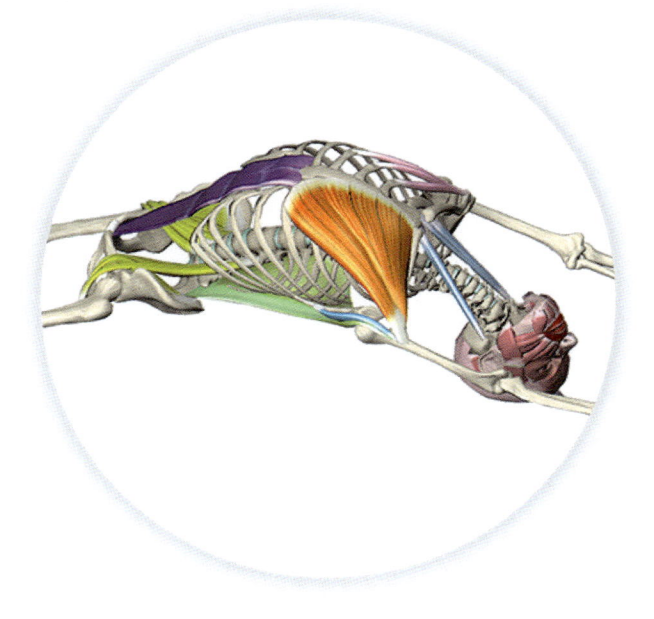

45 Seated Rotation

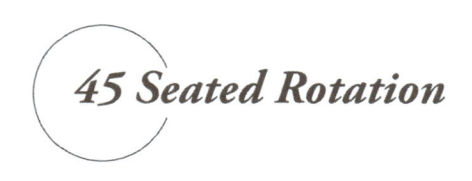

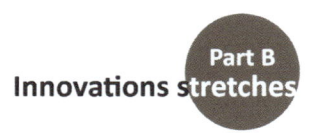

Part B — Innovations stretches

ROTATION
HOW TO STRETCH: Photo A
- Sit on box and rotate shoulders
- Pull shoulder blades together

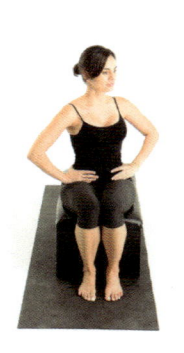

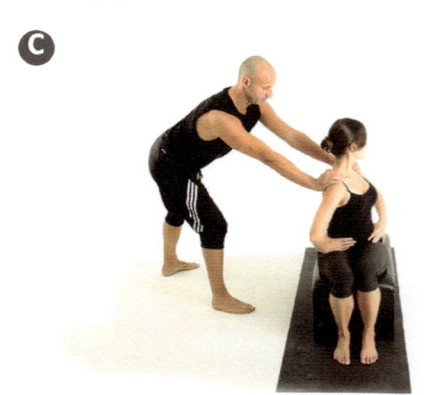

A

HOW TO CONTRACT: Photo B
- Partner to place one hand on back of shoulder, other on front of shoulder
- Try to rotate shoulders back to starting position against standing partner's resistance

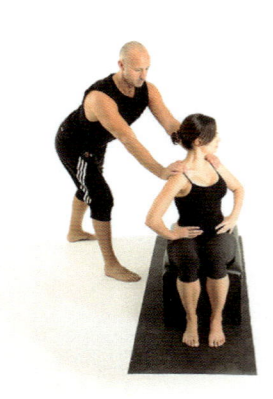

B

HOW TO RESTRETCH: Photo C
- Sit tall and rotate further into stretch
- Partner to assist with rotation
- Keep pelvis neutral

C

Major muscles stretched
- Pectorals
- Obliques abdominals
- Deep spinal rotators

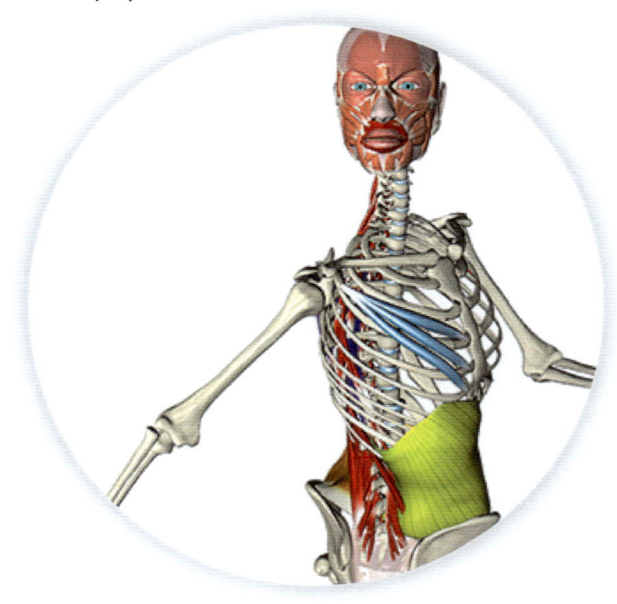

46 Lying Rotation

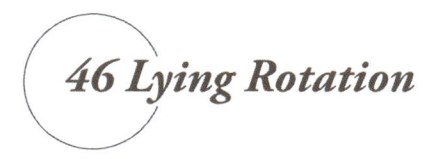

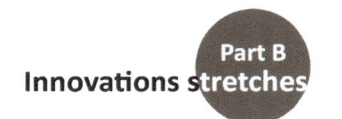

Part B
Innovations stretches

ROTATION

HOW TO SET UP: Photos A and C
- Lie in middle of mat
- Outstretch one arm with hand at head height or higher

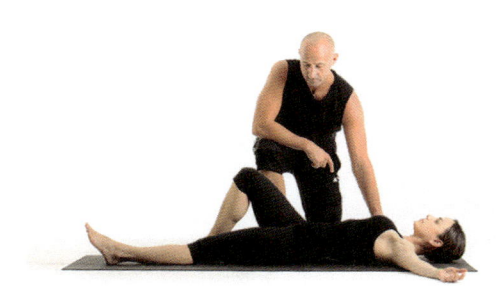

A

HOW TO STRETCH: Photos B and D
- Shift opposite hip to middle of mat
- Rotate pelvis away from outstretched arm
- Keep bottom leg straight
- Allow top leg to drop towards floor

HOW TO CONTRACT: Photos B and D
- Press arm and shoulder up
- Press hip back into partner's hand

HOW TO RESTRETCH: Photos B and D
- Press arm and shoulder into floor
- Allow opposite leg to drop to floor
- Rotate top hip further

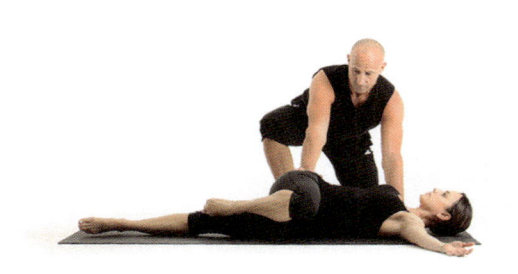

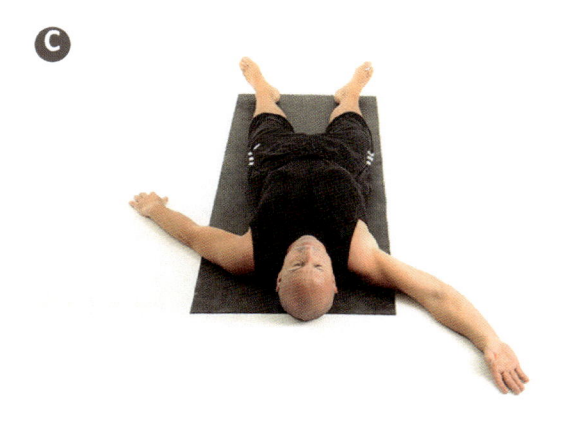

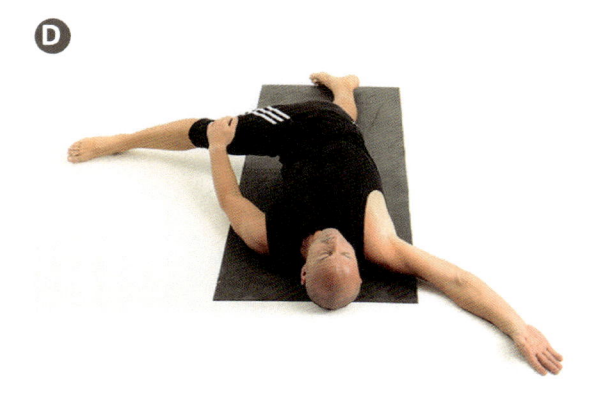

B

C

D

Major muscles stretched
- Pectorals
- Oblique abdominals
- Hip abductors/deep rotators

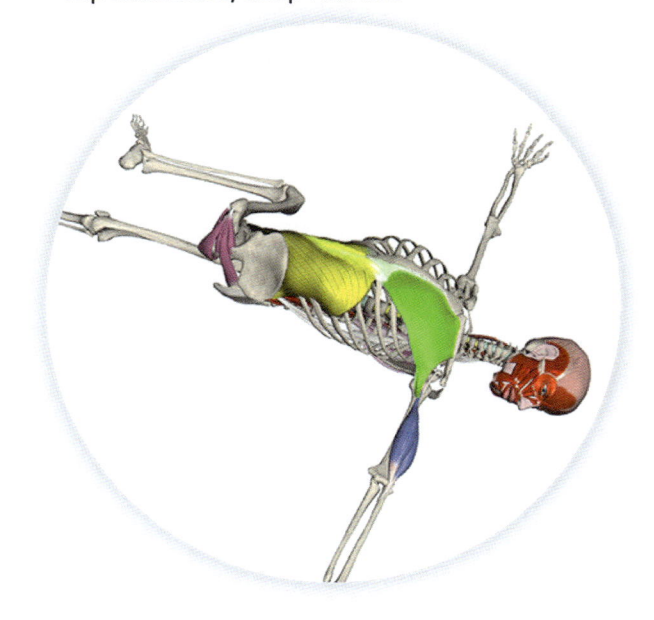

47 Car Crash

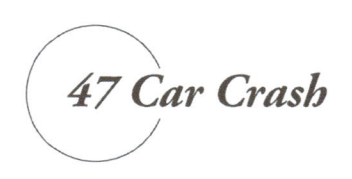

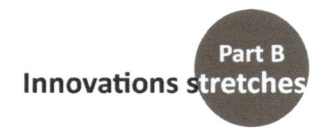

Part B — Innovations stretches

ROTATION

HOW TO SET UP: Photo A
- Sit as pictured with bottom thigh at 90° flexion
- Top leg to remain outstretched

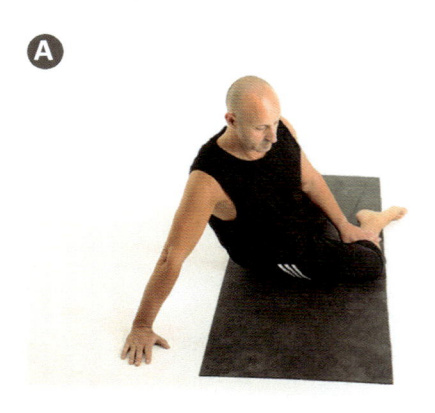

HOW TO STRETCH: Photo B
- Rotate chest above bent leg and lower onto mat as far as comfortable
- Use hands and bent elbows to support chest
- Elongate spine

HOW TO CONTRACT: Photo B
- Use waist muscles to attempt to rotate chest out of the stretch
- Press right hand (in photo) into floor

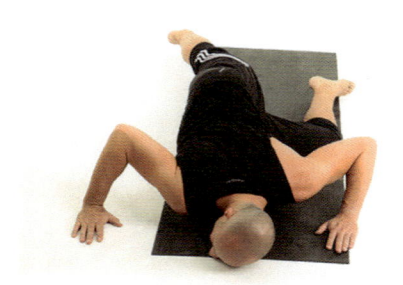

HOW TO RESTRETCH: Photo C
- Rotate shoulders further
- Press top hand into mat to raise shoulder
- Straighten spine

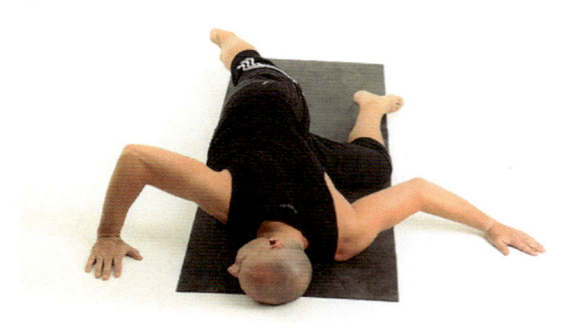

Major muscles stretched
- Oblique abdominals
  Hip abductors
- Deep spinal rotators

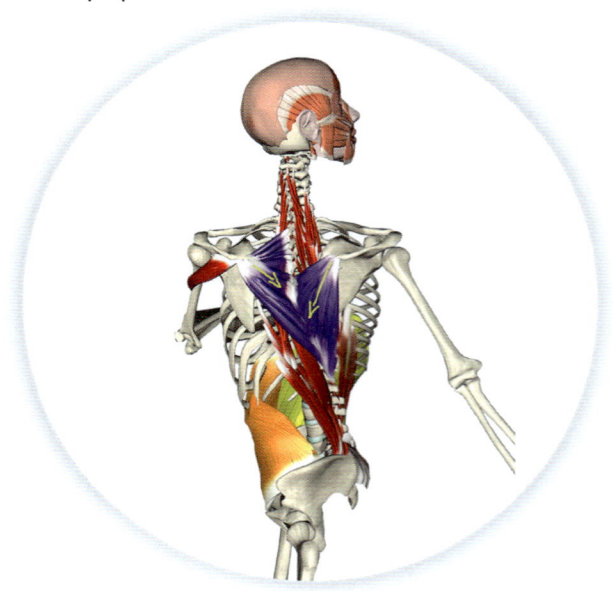

48 Pull and Push

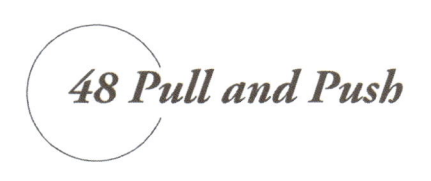

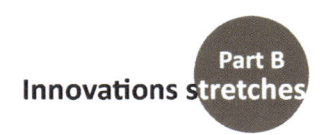

Part B — Innovations stretches

ROTATION

HOW TO SET UP: Photo A
- Kneel parallel to box, at arms length from box, knees below hips

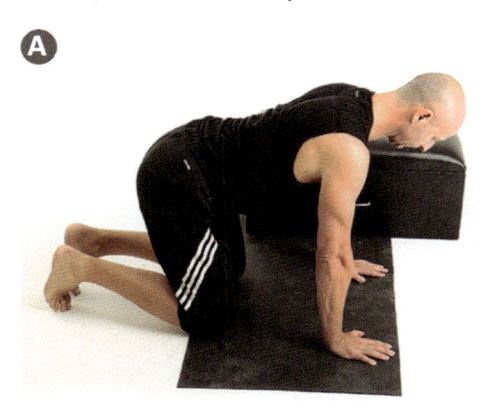

HOW TO RESTRETCH: Photo C
- Lean away from box
- Press top hand into box

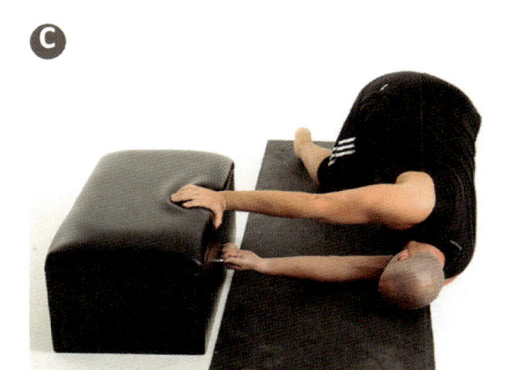

HOW TO STRETCH: Photo B
- Lower chest and reach outside arm under to grasp strap on box
- Place closest arm onto top of box and try to straighten
- Lean away strongly from box

HOW TO CONTRACT: Photo B
- Try to rotate chest back towards mat/floor

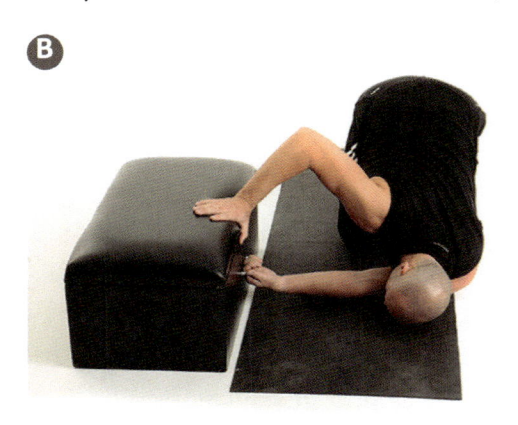

Major muscles stretched
- Levator scapula
- Splenius capitis
- Posterior deltoid
- Middle trapezius
- Rhomboids

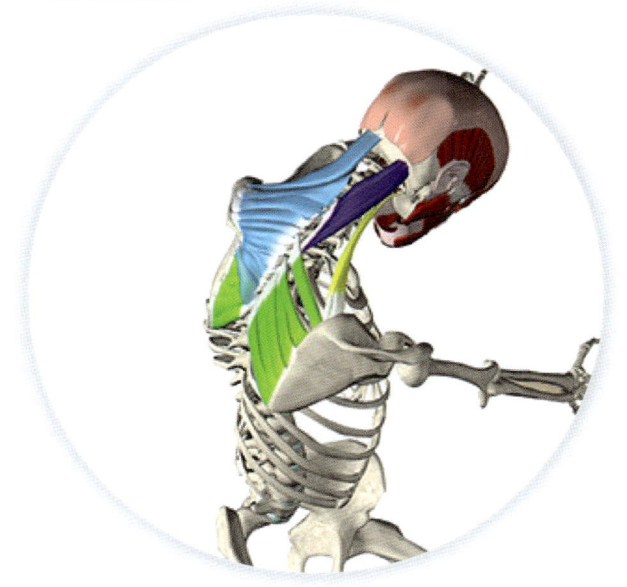

49 Foam Roller Mermaid

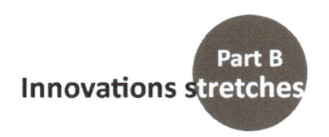

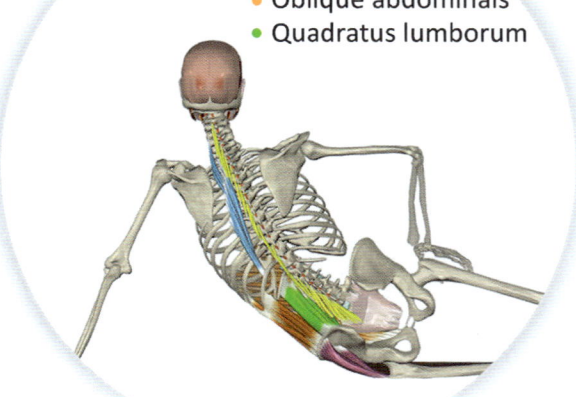

**Part B
Innovations stretches**

LATERAL FLEXION

HOW TO SET UP: Photo A
- Straighten legs and place ankles onto roller
- Balance body on hand and elbow

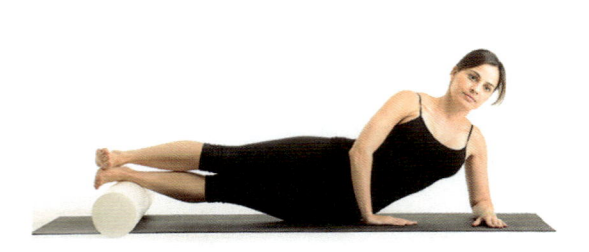

A

HOW TO STRETCH/CONTRACT: Photo B
- Lift chest by pressing arm straight
- Press both feet down into floor

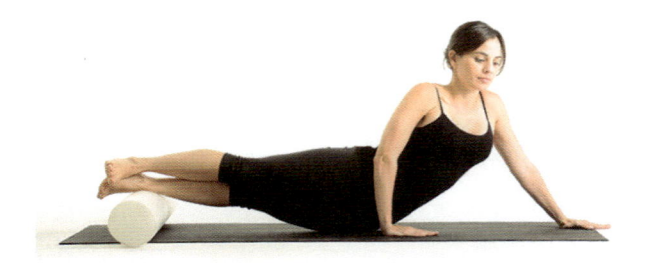

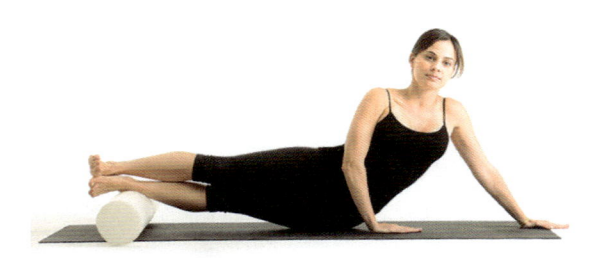

B

HOW TO RESTRETCH: Photo C
- Further straighten both arms
- Move supporting arm closer to body

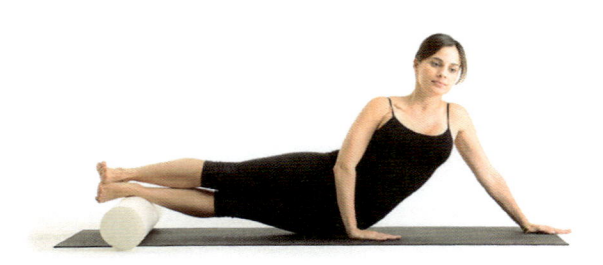

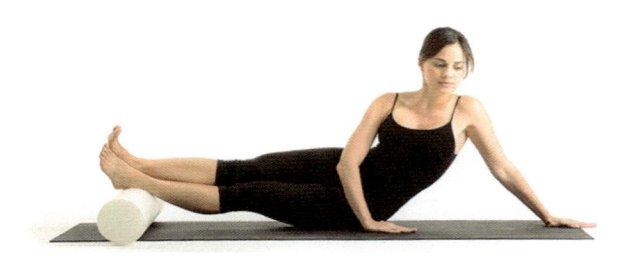

C

VARIATION: Photo D
- Roll top hip forward

D

VARIATION: Photo E
- Roll top hip back

E

Major muscles stretched

- Hip abductors
- Oblique abdominals
- Quadratus lumborum

50 Floor Side Bend

Part B Innovations stretches

LATERAL FLEXION
HOW TO STRETCH: Photo A
- Abduct one leg
- Bend other leg
- Place elbow inside straight leg
- Use arm to pull trunk towards straight leg
- Roll top shoulder backwards above bottom shoulder
- Reach arm overhead
- Partner (if you have one) to press down on hip to keep it anchored to mat
- Partner to press trunk further into side bend

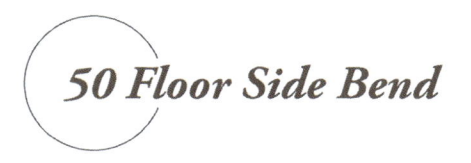

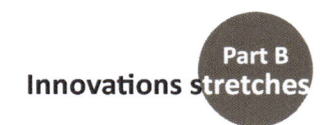

HOW TO CONTRACT: Photo A
- Press shoulders back into partner

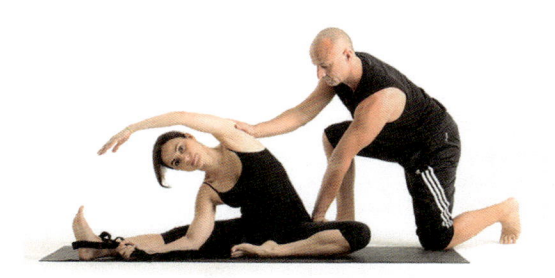

Ⓐ

HOW TO RESTRETCH: Photo B
- Use bottom arm to pull trunk further laterally
- Reach top arm towards foot
- Partner to press hip down and shoulder/spine further sideways

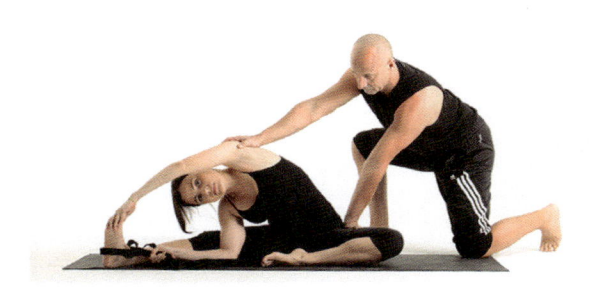

Ⓑ

VARIATION: Photo C
- Bend straight leg and place support underneath
- Bend top arm at elbow

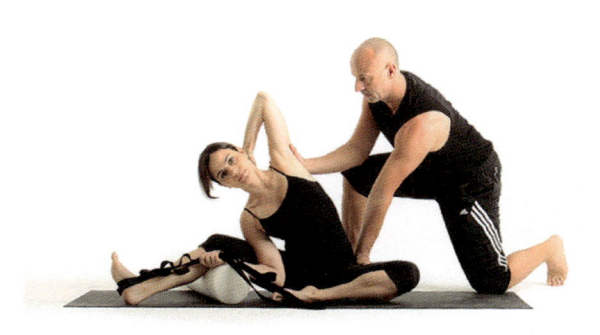

Ⓒ

VARIATION: Photo D
- Roll top shoulder forwards so spine is rotated and bent sideways (lateral flexion)

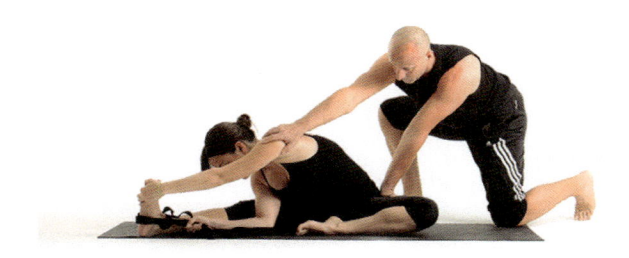

Ⓓ

Major muscles stretched
- Oblique abdominals
- Latissimus dorsi
  Quadratus lumborum

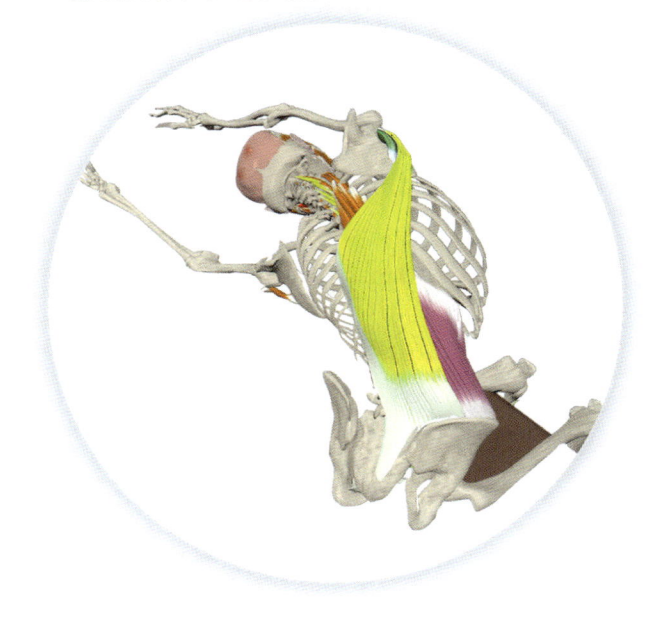

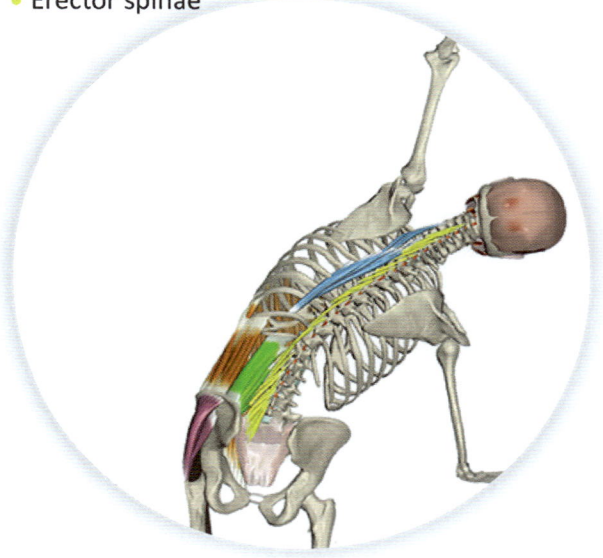

51 Seated Side Bend

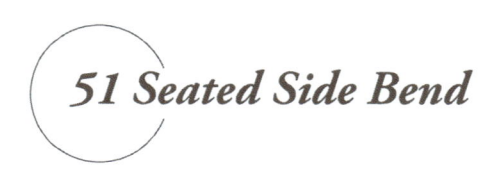

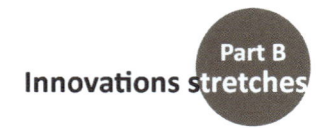

Part B — Innovations stretches

LATERAL FLEXION

HOW TO STRETCH: Photo A
- Sit on box and clasp box strap with hand
- Lean to same side as arm holding box strap
- Reach other arm overhead
- Position top shoulder above bottom one
- Partner to press down on hip and press spine into side bend

HOW TO CONTRACT: Photo A
- Press spine back towards upright position/middle

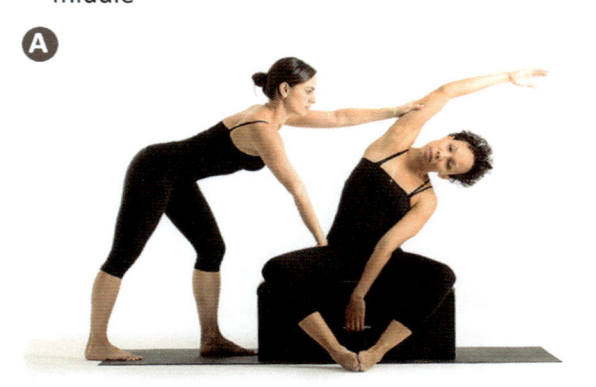

A

HOW TO RESTRETCH: Photo B
- Lean further to side
- Partner to press down on hip and press spine into side bend

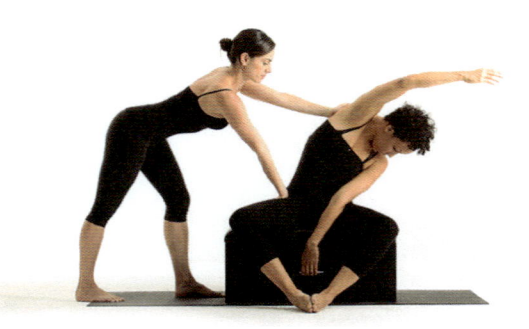

B

VARIATION: Photo C
- Roll top shoulder backwards
- Roll top shoulder forwards (see photo B)

C

Major muscles stretched
- Oblique abdominals
- Quadratus lumborum
  Latissimus dorsi
- Erector spinae

52 Seated Side Bend Variation

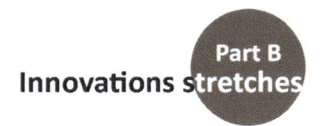

Innovations stretches — Part B

VARIATION: Photo D
- Second partner to pull gently on top arm

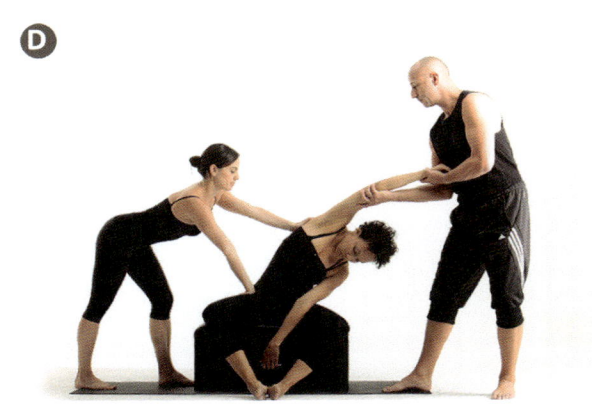

D

VARIATION: Photo E
- Roll top shoulder forward
- Partners to hold hip, press on trunk and pull top arm

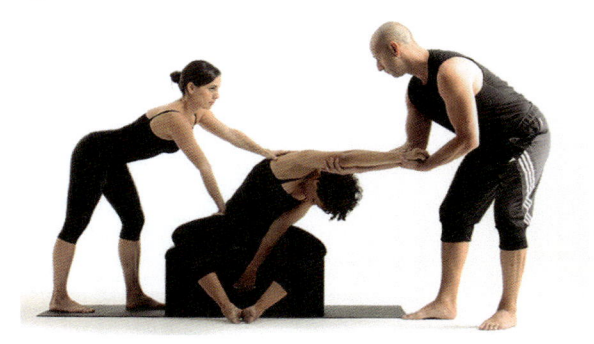

E

Major muscles stretched
- Erector spinae
- Quadratus lumborum
- Internal oblique

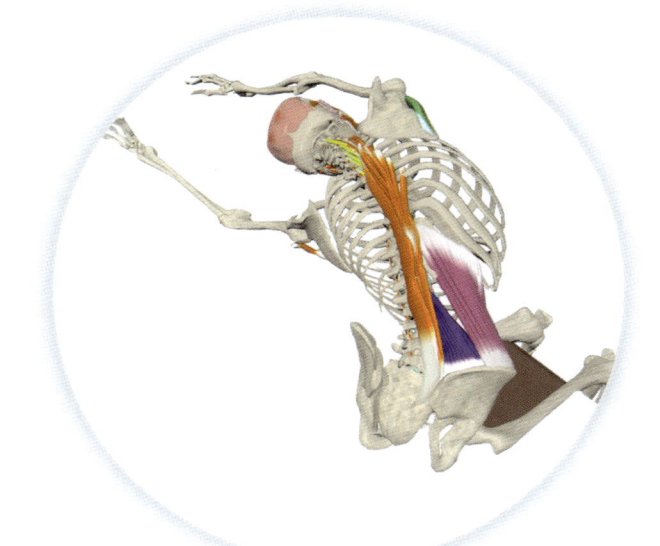

- Latissimus dorsi
- Teres major

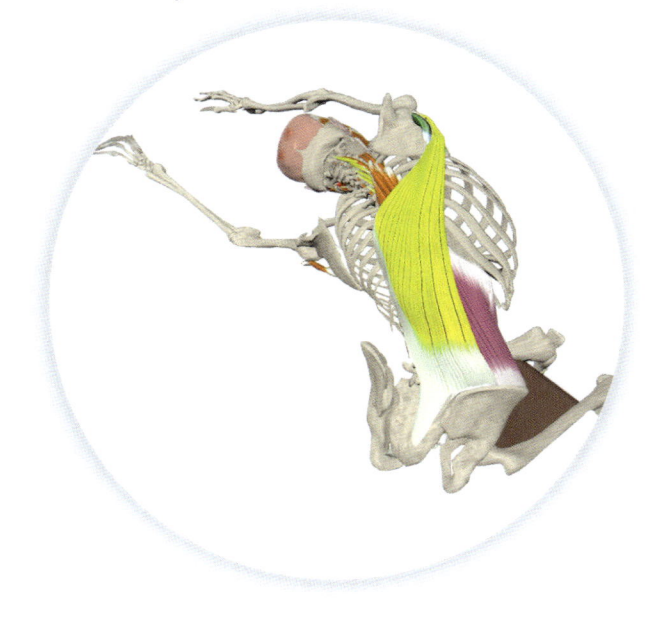

The Chest, Arms and Shoulders
Chapter 7

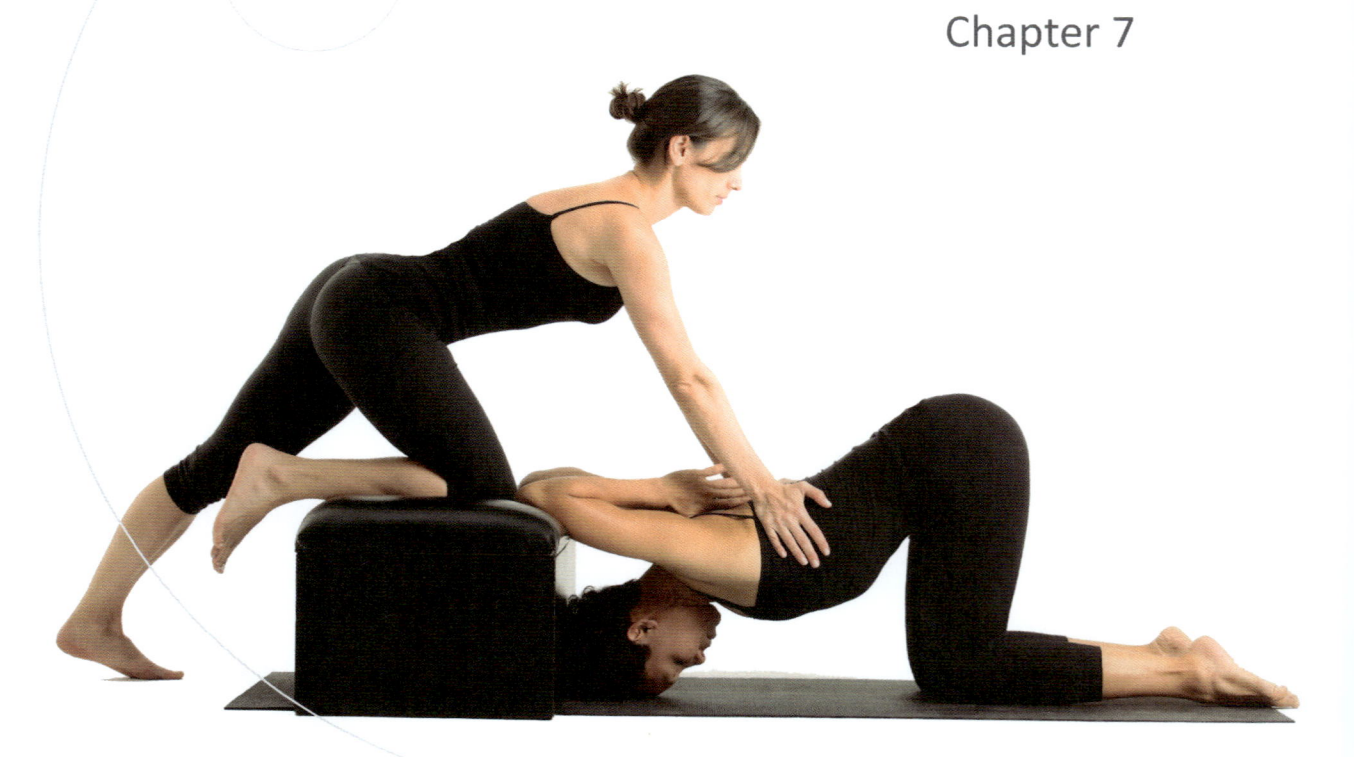

Chapter 7 – Muscle Chart

Arm and Wrist

Muscle	Elbow flexion	Elboe extension	Forearm pronation	Forearm supination	Wrist flexion	Wrist extension	Wrist ulnar deviation	Wrist radial deviation
Bicep brachii	●			●				
Brachialis	●							
Triceps brachii		●						
Anconeus		●						
Brachioradialis	●							
Supinador				●				
Pronator teres			●					
Pronator quadratus			●					
Extensor carpi radialis longus						●		●
Extensor carpi radialis brevis						●		●
Extensor carpi ulnaris						●	●	
Flexor carpi radialis					●			●
Flexor carpi ulnaris					●		●	
Extensor digitorum						●		
Extensor pollicis brevis								●
Extensor pollicis longus				●				●
Abductor pollicis longus								●

Chapter 7 – Muscle Chart

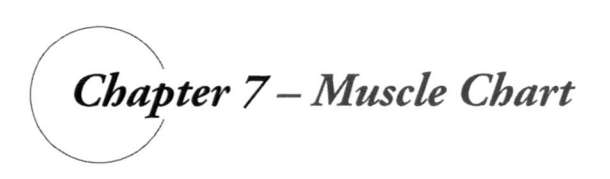

Shoulder

Muscle	Retraction	Protraction	Elevation	Depression	Flexion	Extension	adduction	abduction	Internal rotation	External rotation
Rhomboids	●									
Serratus anterior		●	●					●		
Trapezius	●		●	●			●	●		
Levator scapulae		●	●							
Latissimus dorsi	●			●		●	●		●	
Teres major						●	●		●	
Pectoralis major				●	●		●		●	
Pectoralis minor		●		●						
Anterior deltoid					●				●	
Lateral deltoid								●		
Posterior deltoid						●				●
Supraspinatus								●		
Infraspinatus										●
Teres minor							●			●
Subscapularis									●	
Biceps brachii					●					
Coracobrachialis					●		●			
Triceps brachii						●	●			

Chapter 7 – Muscle Chart

Hand

Muscle	Toe Flexion	Extention	Adduction	Abduction
Flexor digitorum superficialis	●			
Flexor digitorum profundus	●			
Flexor pollicis longus	●			
Flexor pollicis brevis	●			
Flexor digiti minimi brevis	●			
Extensor digitorum		●		
Extensor pollicis longus		●		
Extensor pollicis brevis		●		
Extensor indicis		●		
Extensor digiti minimi		●		
Abductor pollicis longus				●
Abductor pollicis brevis				●
Adductor pollicis			●	
Abductor digiti minimi				●
Lumbricales	●	●		
Dorsal interosseus	●	●	●	

53 Box Lats

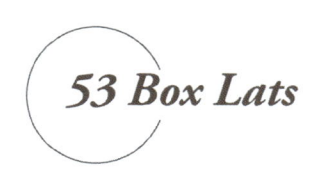

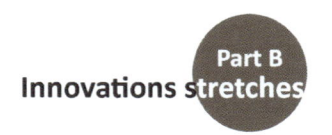

Part B — Innovations stretches

HOW TO STRETCH: Photo A
- Position hips above knees, elbows on box
- Lower chest towards floor

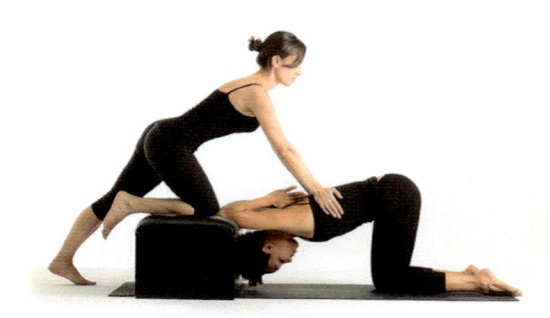

A

HOW TO CONTRACT: Photo B
- Press elbows down into box
- Partner applies downward force onto shoulders

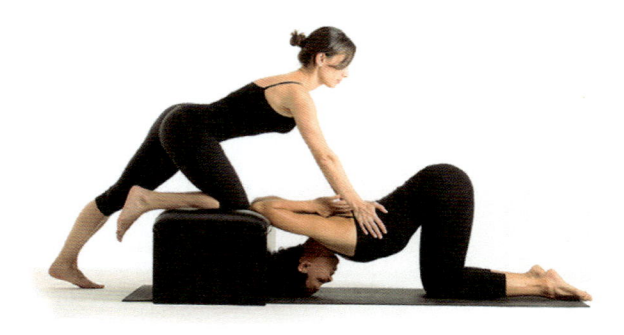

B

HOW TO RESTRETCH: Photo C
- Lower chest further towards floor
- Partner applies force to different parts of spine

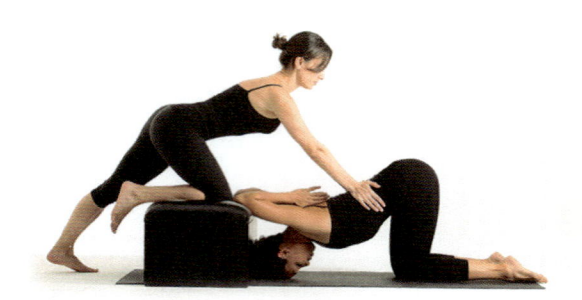

C

VARIATION: Photo D
- Keep hips stable and shift sholders and chest sideways

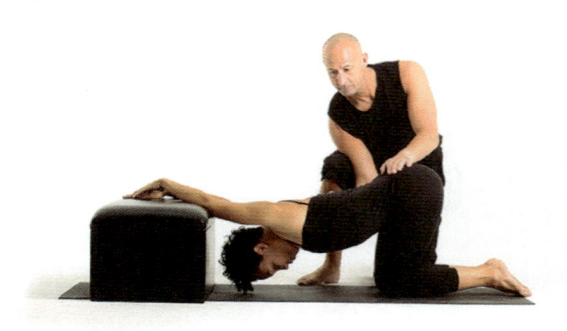

D

Major muscles stretched
- Latissimus dorsi
  Long head of triceps
- Abdominals
  Pectorals

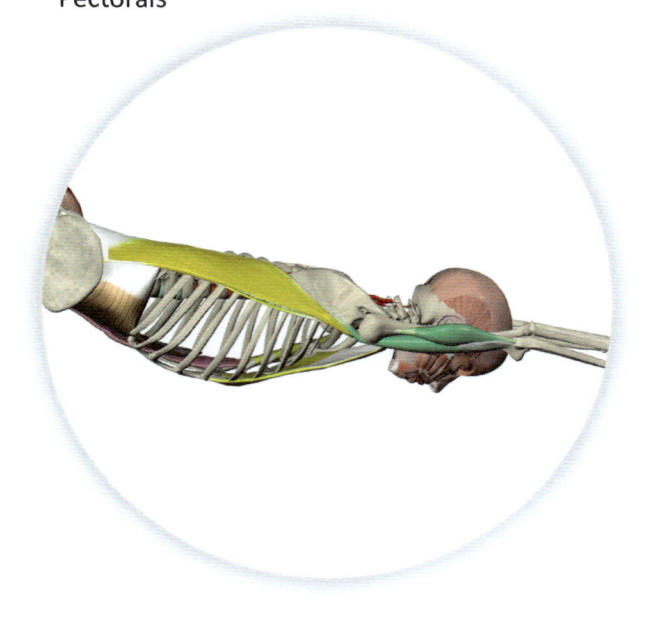

54 Foam Roller Pectoralis Stretch

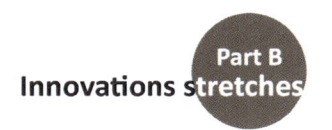

Part B — Innovations stretches

HOW TO STRETCH: Photo A
- Lie on roller with elbow at head height
- Partner to hold elbow onto floor as in Photo B
- Roll chest away from partner

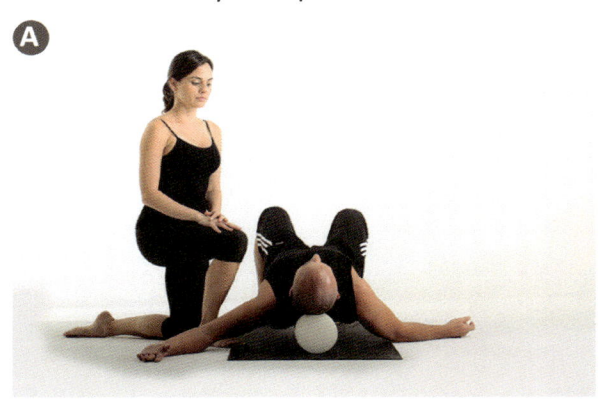

A

HOW TO CONTRACT: Photo B
- Press elbow up into partner

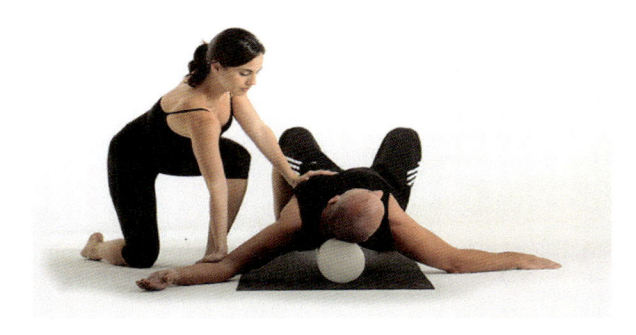

B

HOW TO RESTRETCH: Photo C
- Roll chest and head further from partner

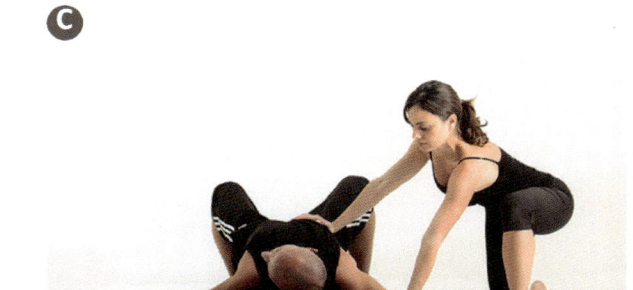

C

VARIATION: Photo D
- To stretch different pectoralis major fibres, repeat entire sequence with arm being stretched positioned lower and higher in relation to head

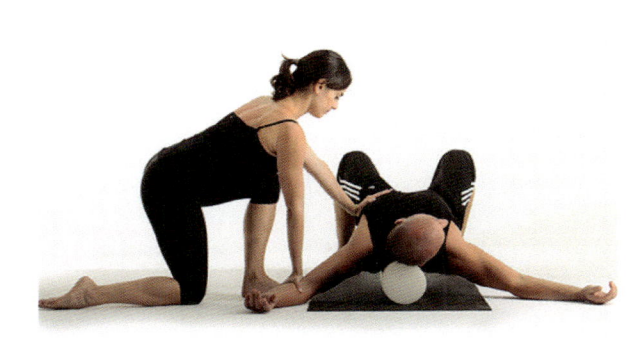

D

Major muscles stretched
- Pectorals

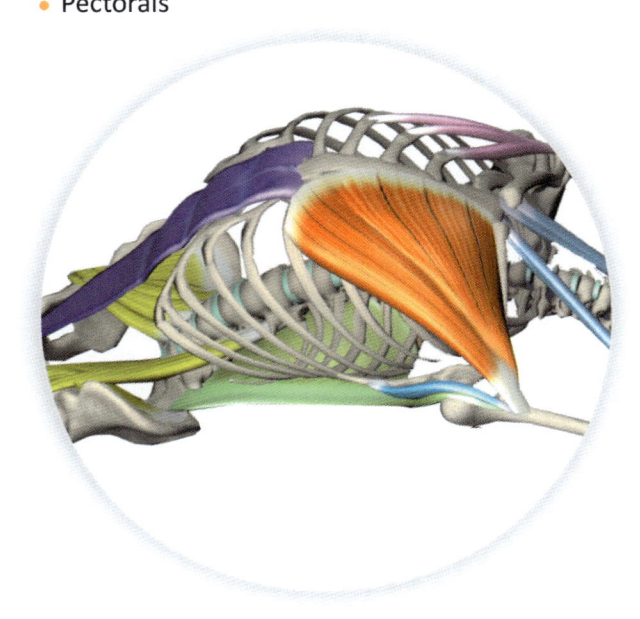

55 Lying Pectoralis Major

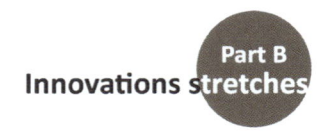

Part B
Innovations stretches

HOW TO STRETCH: Photo A
- Lie as pictured with elbow at head height
- Keep front of shoulder on mat
- Roll opposite shoulder, hip and leg backwards
- Press opposite hand down into floor

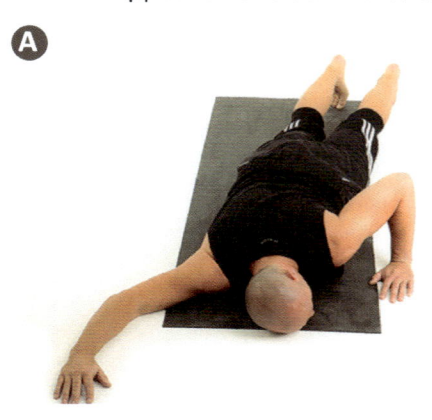

A

HOW TO CONTRACT: Photo B
- Press arm under stretch into floor

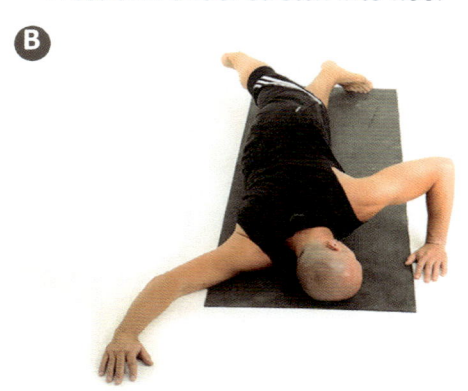

B

HOW TO RESTRETCH: Photo C
- Roll hip and leg back further
- Press opposite hand down into floor

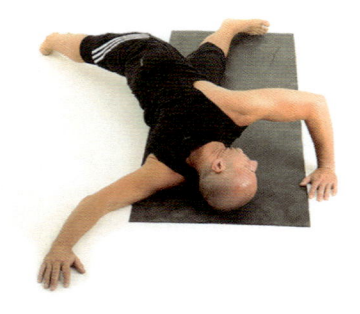

C

Major muscles stretched
- Pectorals

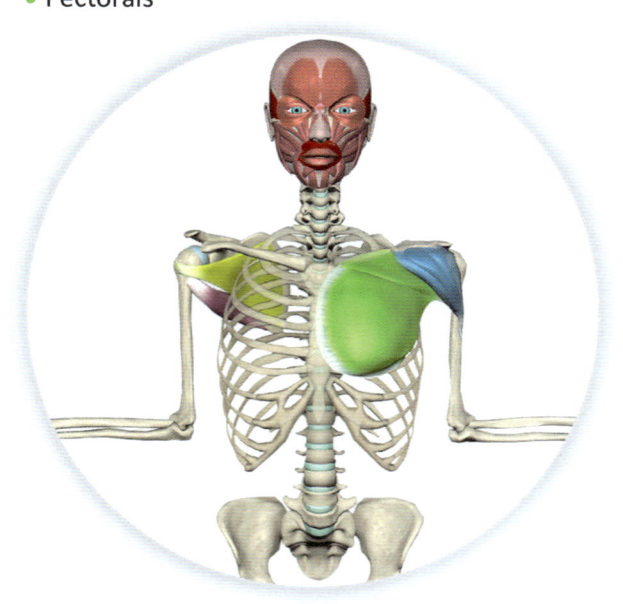

56 Lying Bicep

Part B
Innovations stretches

HOW TO STRETCH: Photo A
- Place forearm and front of shoulder onto floor (forearm pronated, shoulder neutral if possible)
- Hand of straight arm to be higher than head
- Roll opposite hip, shoulder and leg backwards
- Press opposite hand into floor

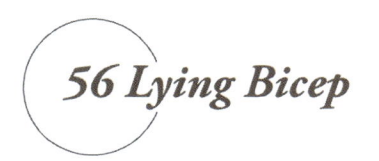

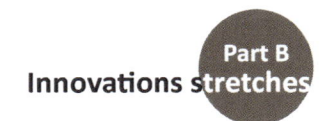

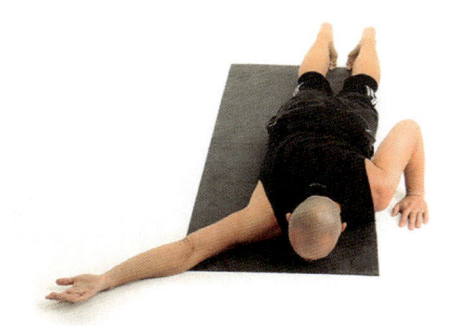

HOW TO CONTRACT: Photo B
- Press arm down into floor

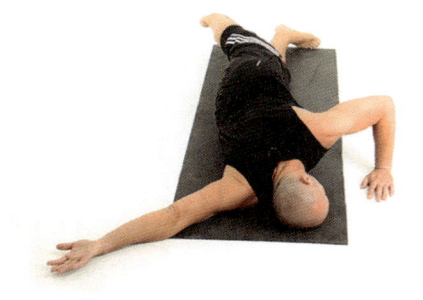

HOW TO RESTRETCH: Photo C and D
- Roll opposite hip, leg and shoulder further back
- Press opposite hand into floor
- Make a fist and flex wrist for greater forearm stretch

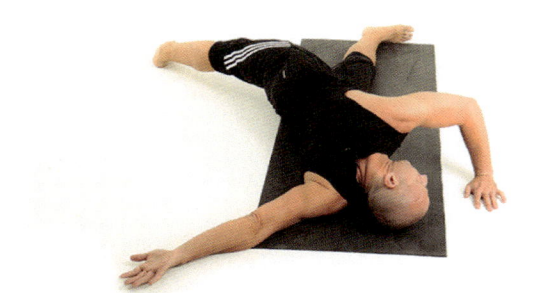

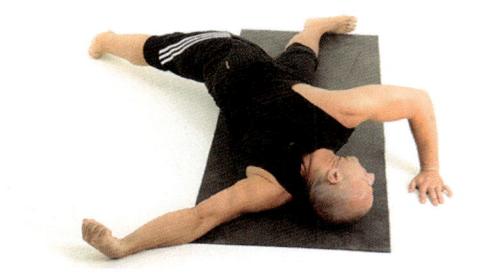

Major muscles stretched
Anterior deltoid
- Biceps brachi
Brachialis
Forearm extensors

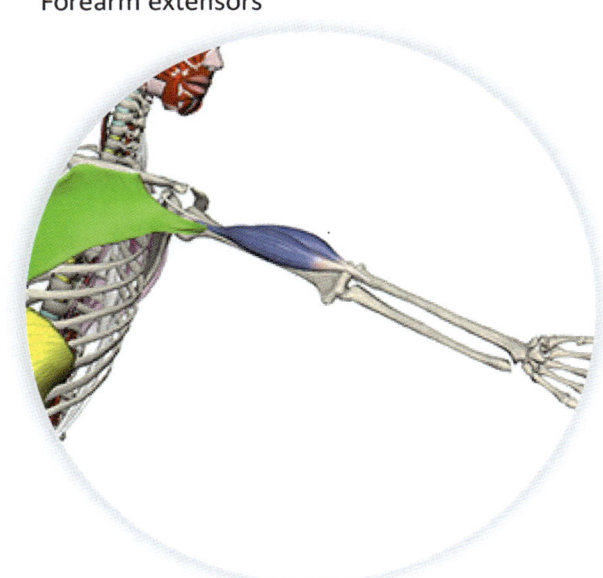

57 Standing Pectoralis Minor

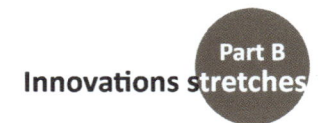

Part B
Innovations stretches

HOW TO STRETCH: Photo A
- Partner draws shoulder blade back towards spine (retraction)
- Partner places one hand on scapula to press it against rib cage
- Partner places other hand on front of shoulder
- Person being stretched turns chest away from hand on front of shoulder

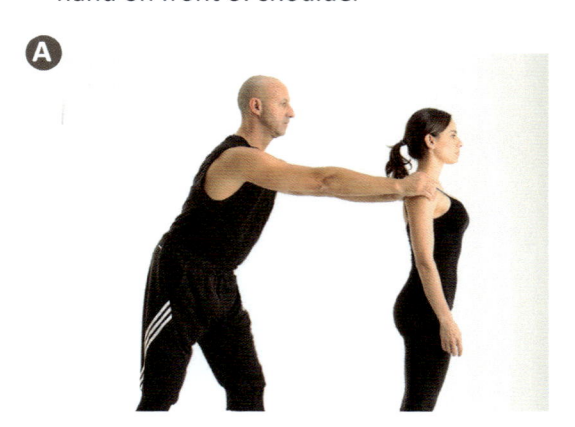

A

HOW TO CONTRACT: Photo B
- Person being stretched presses front of shoulder into partner's hand

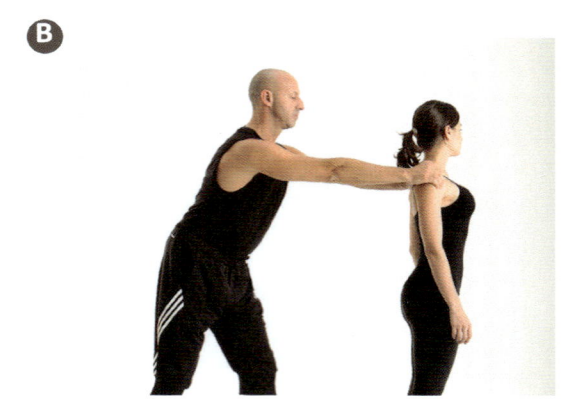

B

HOW TO RESTRETCH: Photo C
- Turn chest further from partner's hand

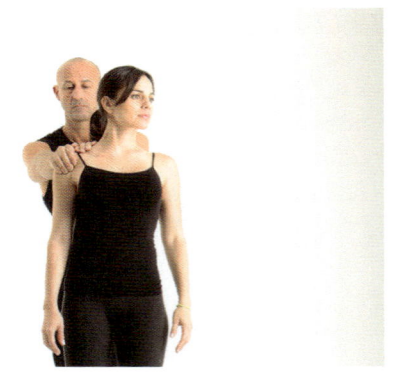

C

VARIATION: Photo D
- To stretch both sides at once, clasp fingers together or hold a strap
- Rotate chest from tight side

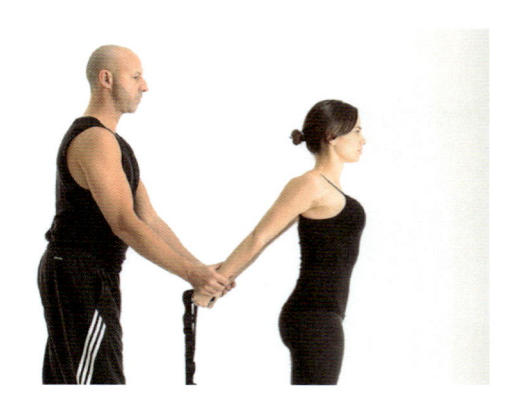

D

Major muscles stretched
- Pectoralis minor
  Serratus anterior

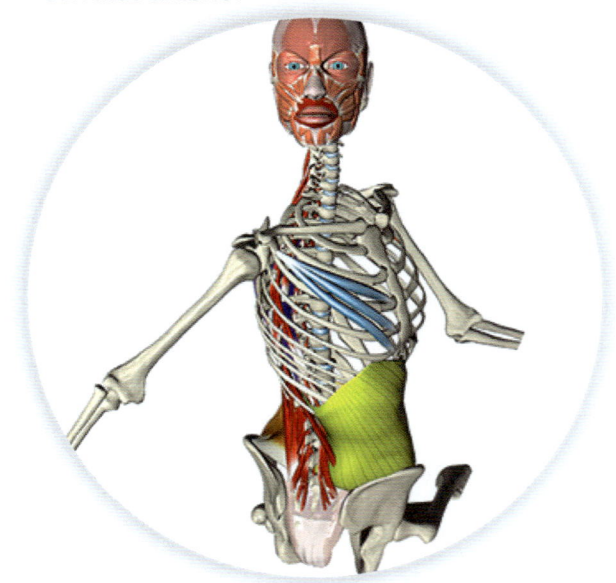

58 Tricep/Lats

Innovations stretches — Part B

HOW TO STRETCH: Photo A
- Reach hand between shoulder blades
- Pull elbow towards back of head

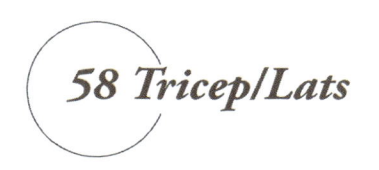

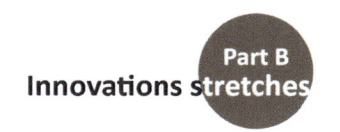

HOW TO CONTRACT: Photo A
- Press elbow away from body

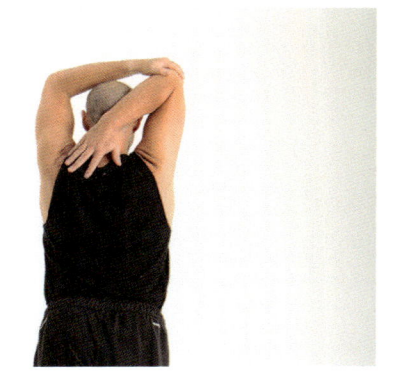

A

HOW TO RESTRETCH: Photo B
- Pull elbow further towards back of head

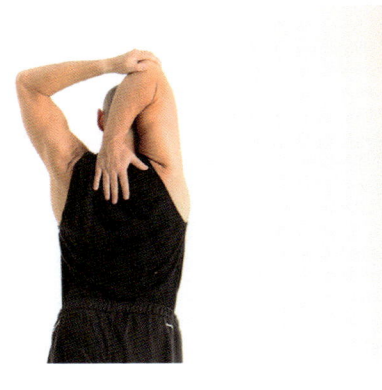

B

Major muscles stretched
- Triceps
- Latissimus dorsi

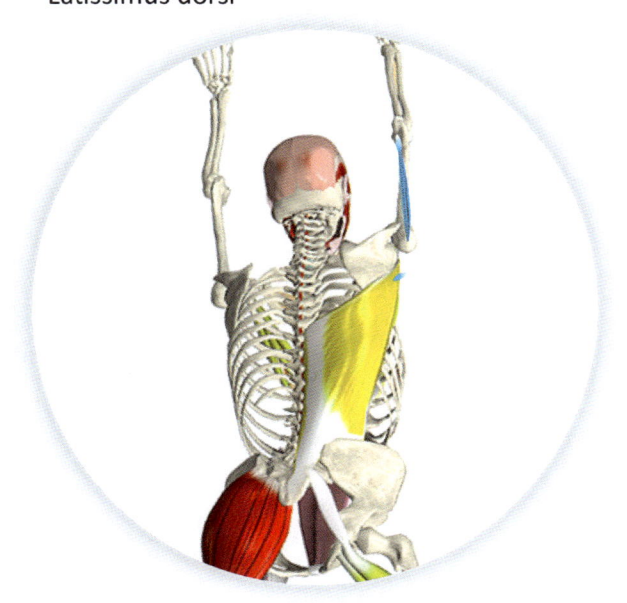

59 Partner Internal Rotators

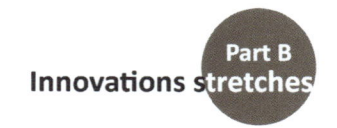

Part B
Innovations stretches

HOW TO STRETCH: Photo A
- Bend arm to 90°
- Fix elbow in towards side of body and draw hand backwards

HOW TO CONTRACT: Photo A
- Press hand forward towards front of body

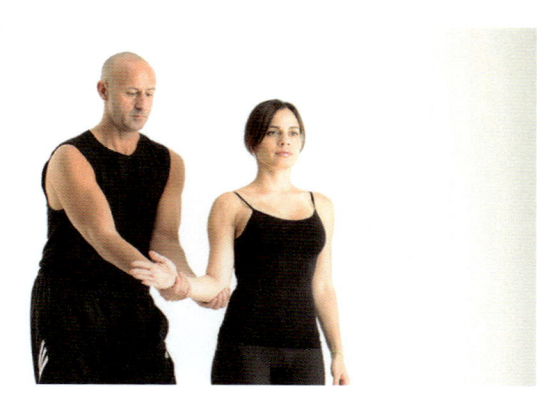

A

HOW TO RESTRETCH: Photo B
- Take hand backwards and keep elbow stationary

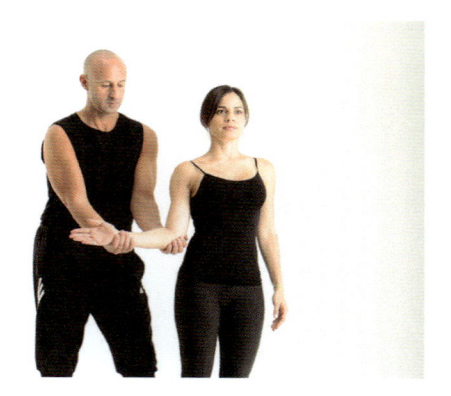

B

Major muscles stretched
- Teres major
- Subscapularis

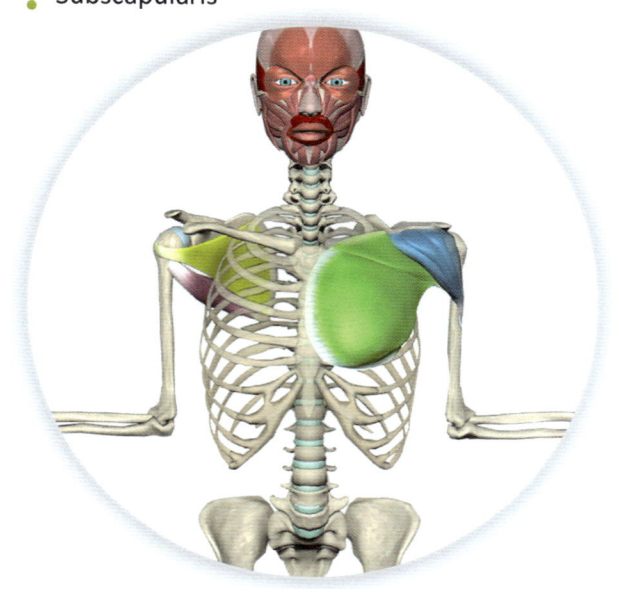

60 Partner External Rotators

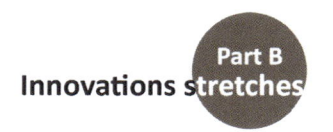

Part B — Innovations stretches

HOW TO STRETCH: Photo A
- Place hand behind back
- Bend elbow to 90°
- Pull scapula towards spine
- Partner to stabilise shoulder and draw hand away from body

HOW TO CONTRACT: Photo A
- Press hand back towards body

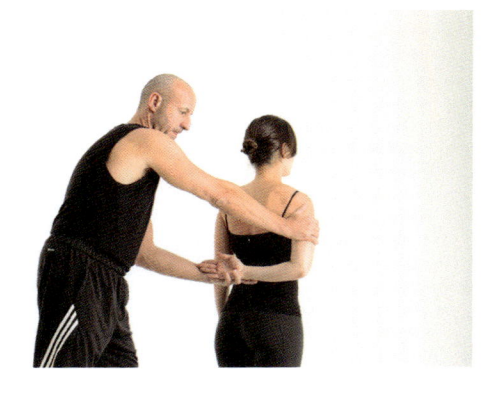

HOW TO RESTRETCH: Photo B
- Stabilise shoulder
- Keep scapula pulled back towards spine
- Draw hand further away from spine

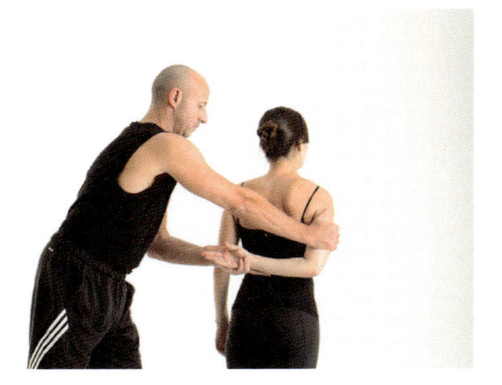

Major muscles stretched
- Infraspinatus
- Posterior deltoid
- Teres minor

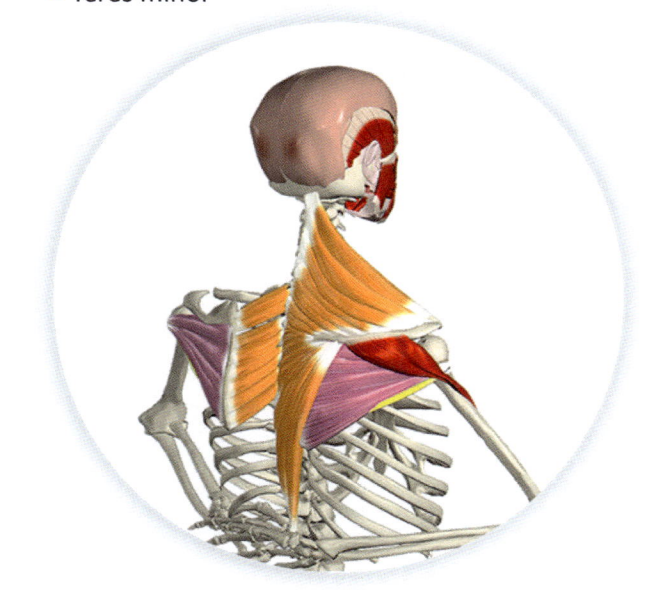

61 Stick Internal Rotators

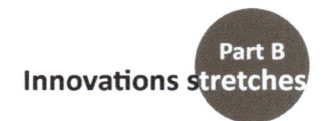

Part B
Innovations stretches

HOW TO STRETCH: Photo A
- Place arm in front of body with elbow at shoulder height
- Bend elbow to 90°
- Place stick on outside of forearm
- Pull on lower part of stick towards centre of body, as in Photo C

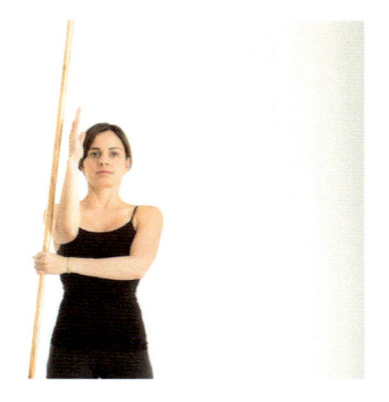

A

HOW TO CONTRACT: Photo B
- Press hand being stretched back towards start position

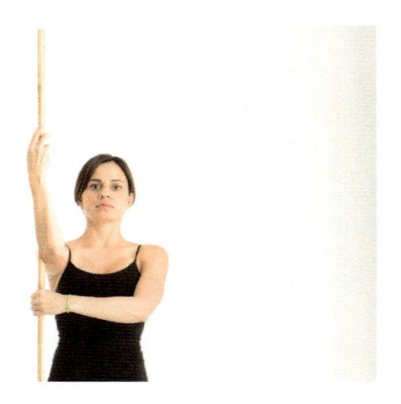

B

HOW TO RESTRETCH: Photo C
- Pull on stick with lower hand, pulling in upward direction

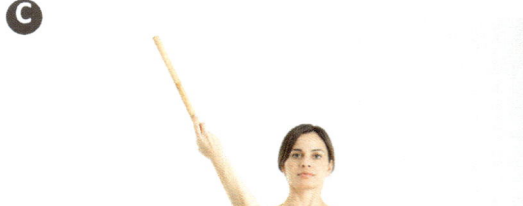

C

Major muscles stretched
- Teres major
- Subscapularis

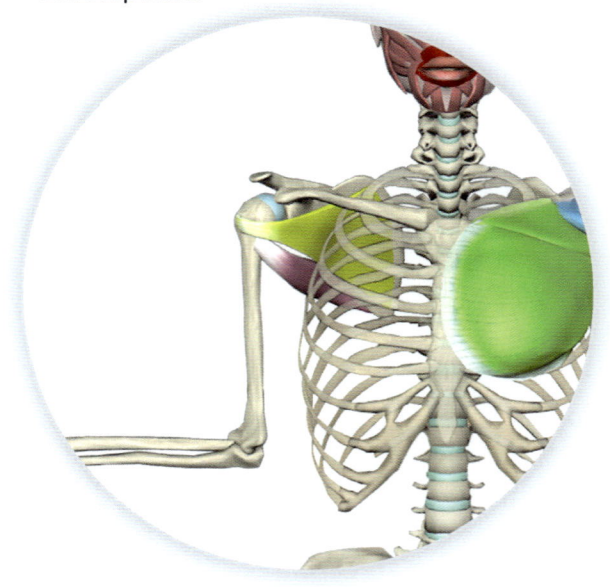

62 Forearm Extensors

Part B Innovations stretches

HOW TO STRETCH: Photo A
- Kneel on floor placing backs of hands onto floor
- Lean weight into hands and backwards

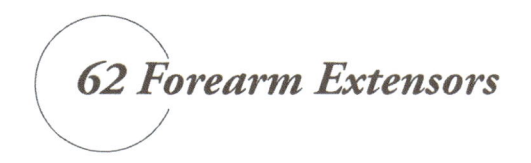

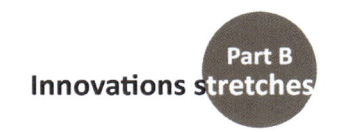

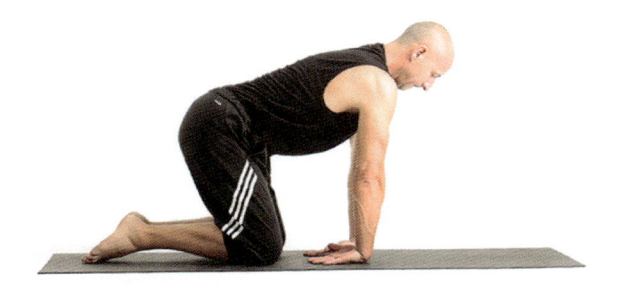

A

HOW TO CONTRACT: Photo B
- Press back of hands down into floor

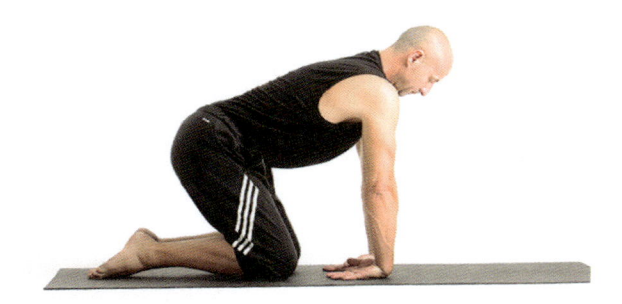

B

HOW TO RESTRETCH: Photo B
- Press more weight down onto wrists/hands and lean back further

Major muscles stretched
Forearm extensors

63 Forearm Flexors

Part B
Innovations stretches

HOW TO STRETCH: Photo A
- Kneel on floor and place palms onto floor
- Fingers must point back towards knees
- Lean bodyweight backwards

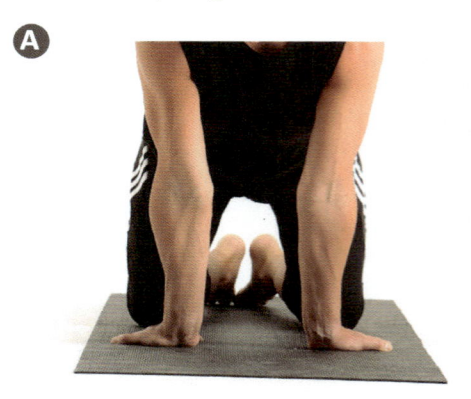

A

VARIATIONS: Photos B and C
- Lean weight above each finger in turn

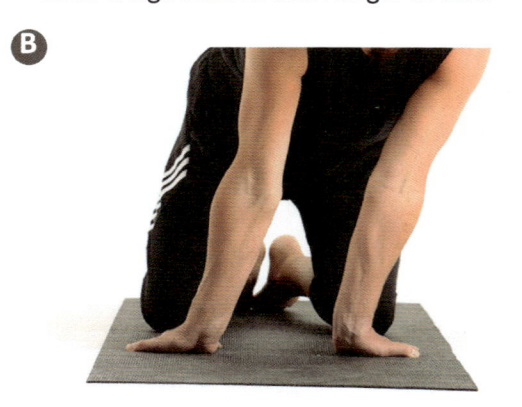

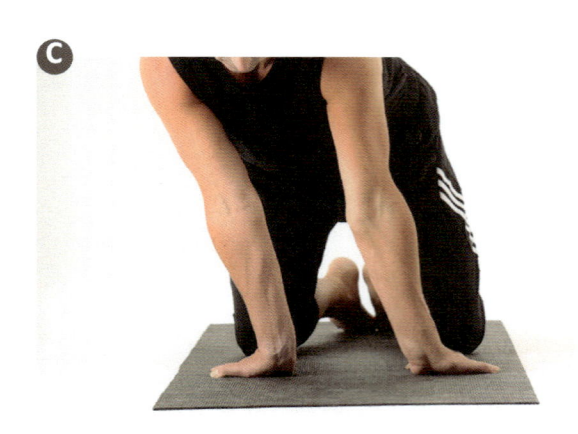

B

C

HOW TO CONTRACT: Photo D
- Press both hands into floor

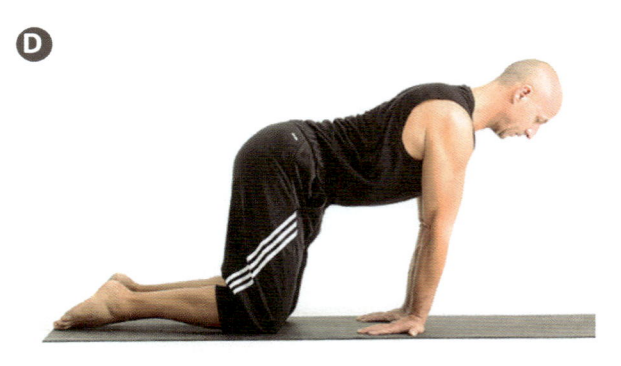

D

HOW TO RESTRETCH: Photo E
- Lean backwards and repeat variations

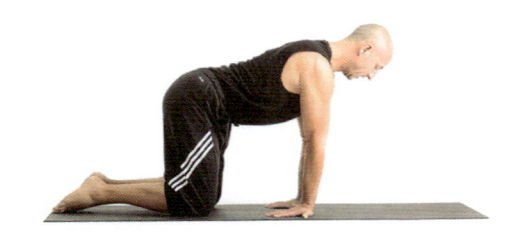

E

Major muscles stretched
Forearm flexors

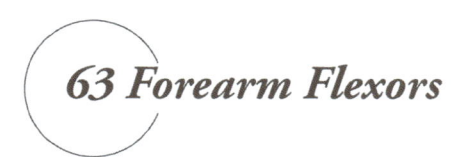

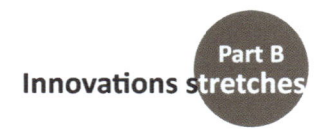

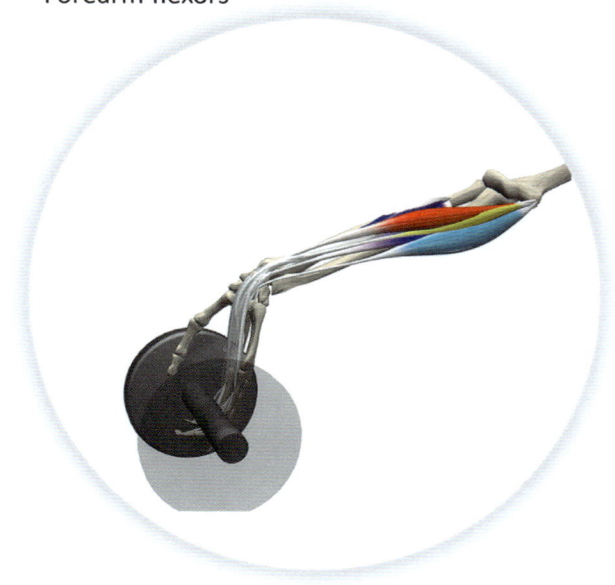

64 Pronators

Part B
Innovations stretches

HOW TO STRETCH: Photo A
- Straighten arm in front of body
- Flex hand at wrist and press wrist further into flexion with other hand
- Turn fingers away from centre of body
- Turn arm outwards (external rotation)

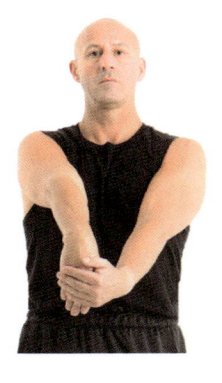

A

HOW TO CONTRACT: Photo B
- Press fingers back towards centre of body

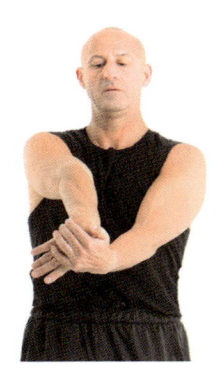

B

Major muscles stretched
Forearm extensors
Pronators

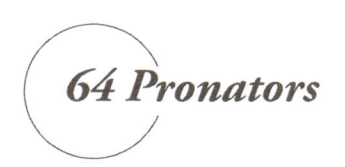

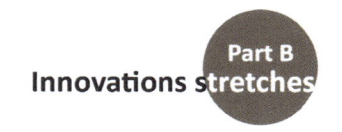

HOW TO RESTRETCH: Photo C
- Repeat instructions for photo A

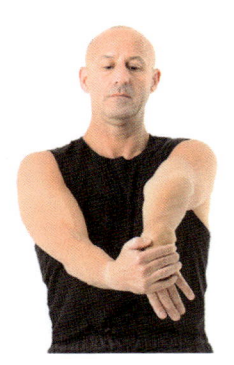

C

The Neck
Chapter 8

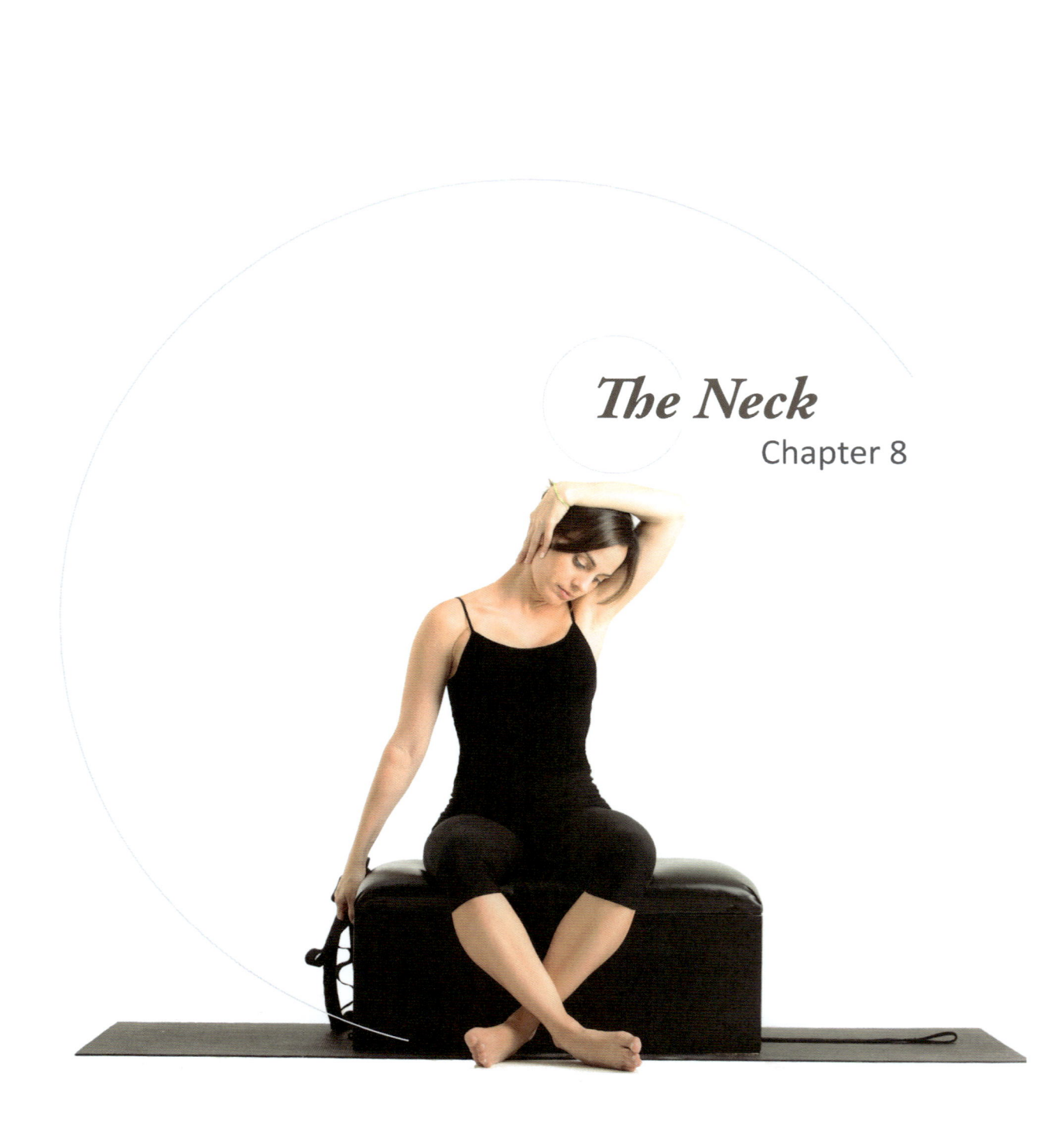

Chapter 8 – Muscle Chart

Neck

Muscle	Flexion	Extension	Lateral flexion	Lateral extension	Rotation
Semispinalis capitis		●	●	●	●
Splenius capitis		●	●	●	●
Sternocleidomastoid	●		●	●	●
Levator scapulae		●	●	●	
Trapezius		●	●	●	●

66 Neck Flexion

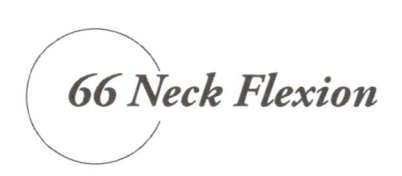

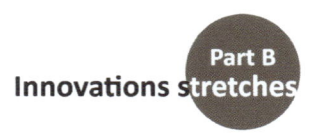

**Part B
Innovations stretches**

HOW TO STRETCH: Photo A
- Tuck chin towards neck; i.e. nod the head
- Take chin towards chest

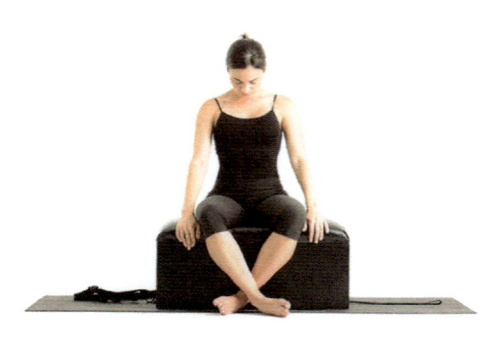

A

HOW TO CONTRACT: Photo B
- Place hands onto back of head
- Take as much weight onto head as is comfortable
- Press head back into hands

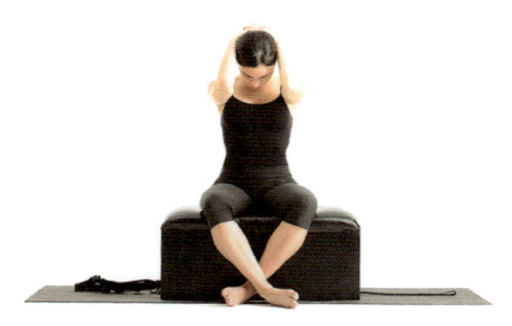

B

HOW TO RESTRETCH: Photo C
- Take chin further to neck
- Take chin further to chest

VARIATION: Photo C
- Turn face towards both armpits
- If turning to right, press with right hand onto head then repeat on other side

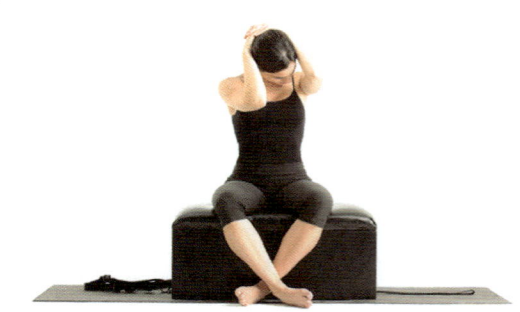

C

Major muscles stretched
- Suboccipitals

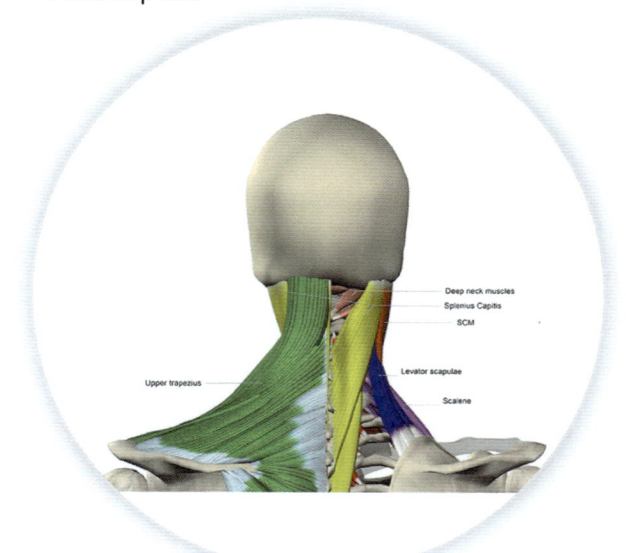

67 Neck Flexion and Rotation

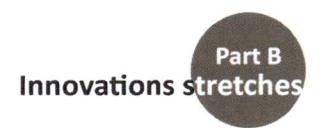

Innovations stretches — Part B

HOW TO STRETCH: Photos A and B
- Place hand behind hip on corner of box
- Relax shoulders and lean away from hand
- Take chin towards chest and turn face to one shoulder
- Reach opposite hand and place it over head
- Rest head onto arm and shoulder

HOW TO CONTRACT: Photo C
- Press head back towards rear arm/hand

HOW TO RESTRETCH: Photo C
- Take chin further to chest and turn face further to armpit

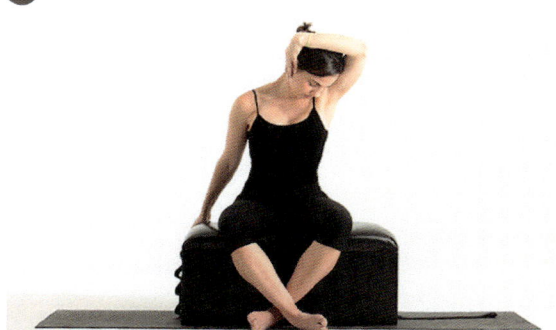

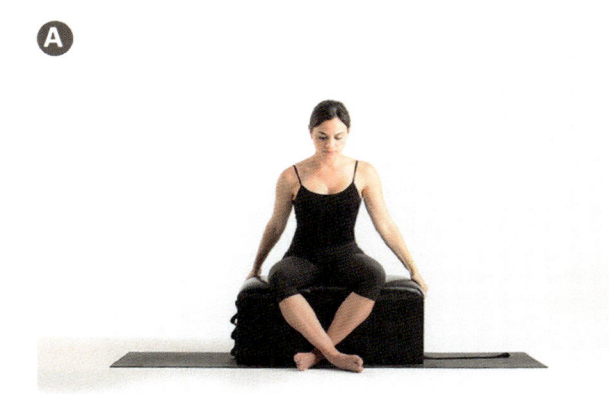

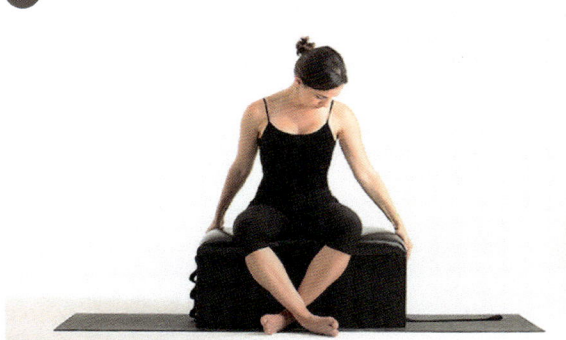

Major muscles stretched
- Levator scapula
- Upper trapezius

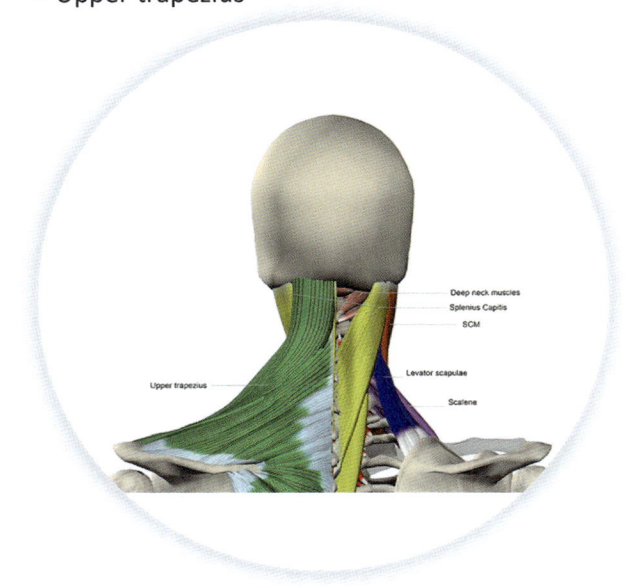

68 Neck Lateral Flexion

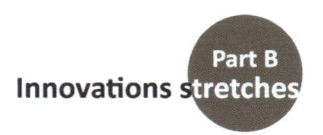

Part B
Innovations stretches

HOW TO STRETCH: Photos A and B
- Place arm alongside hip, in line with shoulder
- Clasp box or strap
- Lean away from arm and take head towards opposite shoulder
- Reach opposite arm over head
- Rest head onto opposite arm or shoulder

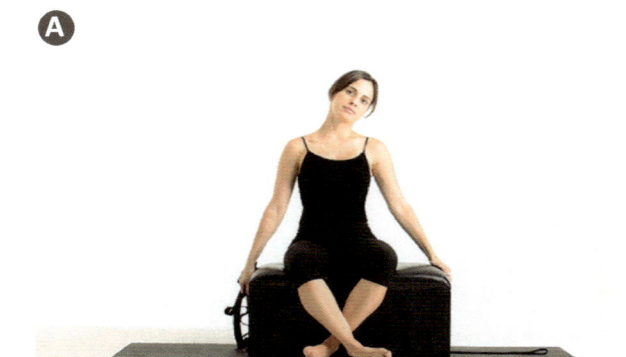

HOW TO RESTRETCH: Photo C
- Take head further towards opposite shoulder
- Rest head onto shoulder/arm
- Use finger to pull lightly on head
- Turn face towards armpit

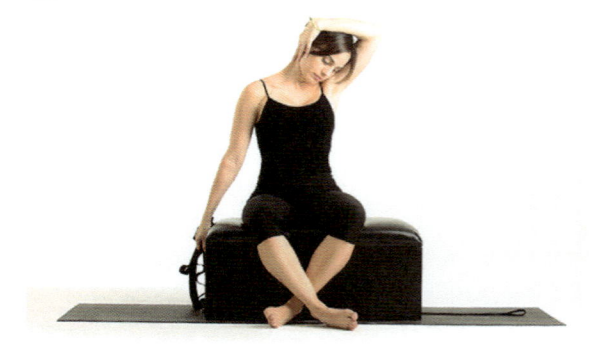

A

C

HOW TO CONTRACT: Photo B
- Press head back towards start position/centre

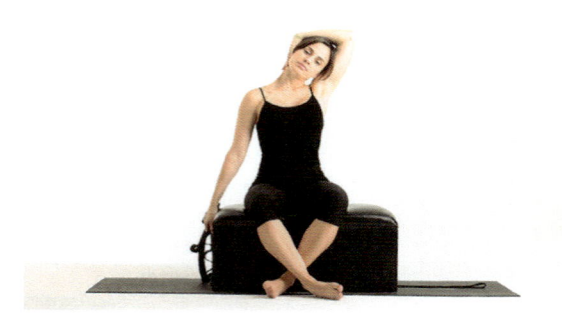

B

Major muscles stretched
- Scalenus medius and posterior
- Upper trapezius

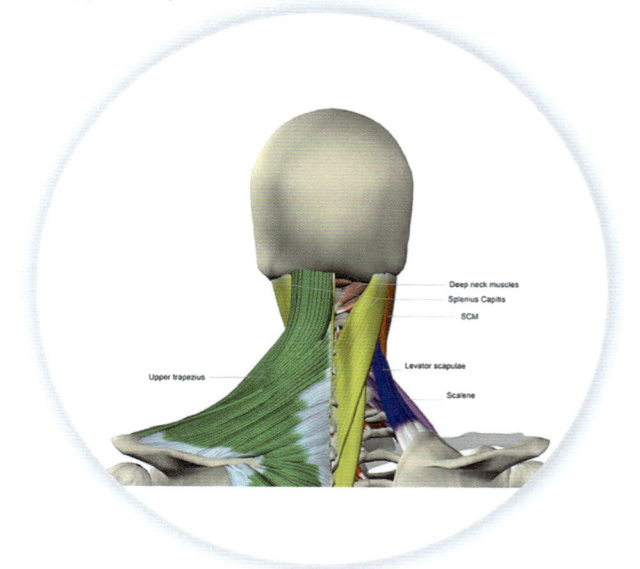

69 Neck Rotation

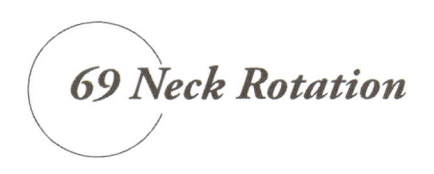

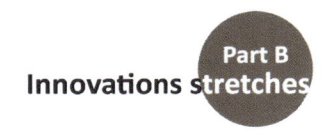

Part B
Innovations stretches

HOW TO STRETCH: Photos A and B
- Turn face towards shoulder
- Prevent shoulders from moving
- Place hand onto side of face. If turning to left, use left hand

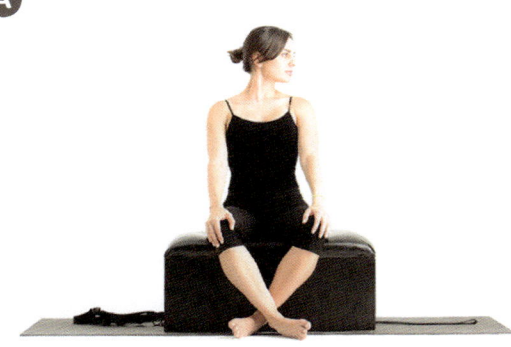

A

Major muscles stretched
- SCM
- Splenius
- Levator scapulae

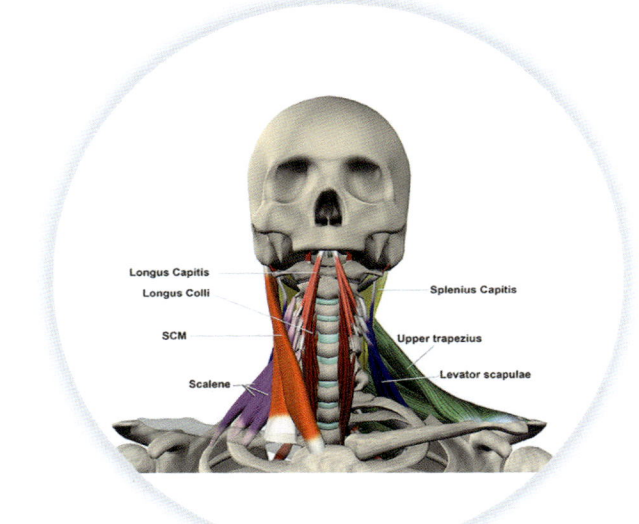

HOW TO CONTRACT: Photo B
- Press head back towards centre/hand

HOW TO RESTRETCH: Photos B and C
- Turn face further from centre

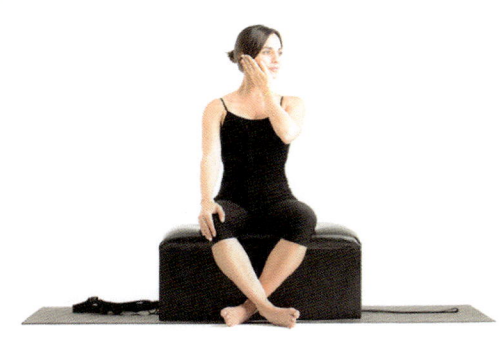

B

Deep neck muscles
- Upper trapezius
- Levator scapulae

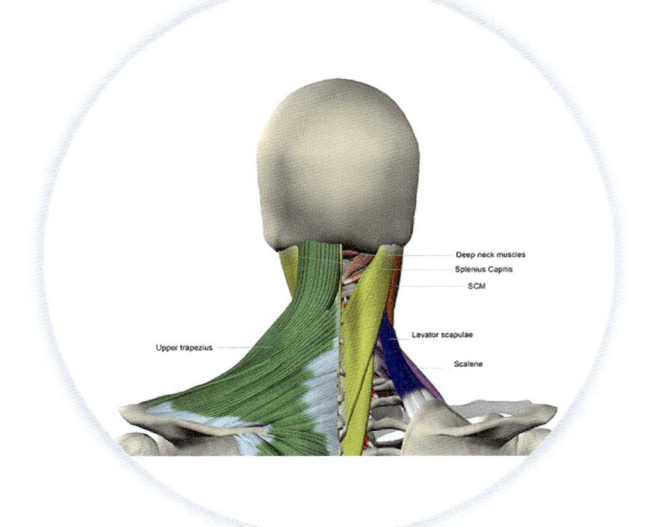

VARIATION: Photo C
- Turn face and nod head

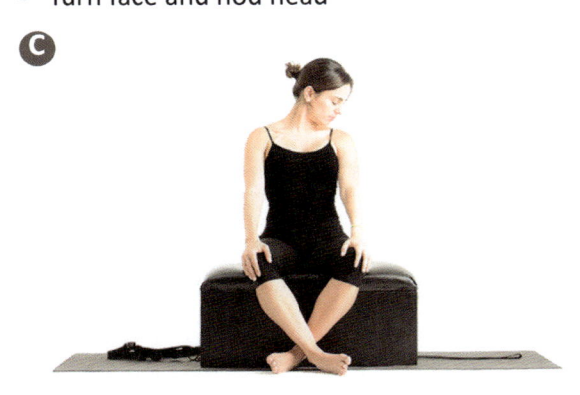

C

70 Neck Extension and Rotation

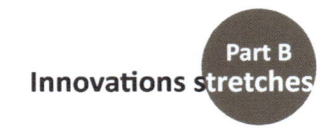

Part B
Innovations stretches

HOW TO STRETCH: Photos A and B
- Place one hand in front of hip, level with knee
- Clasp corner of box or strap with this hand
- Take head backwards and turn face away from front hand

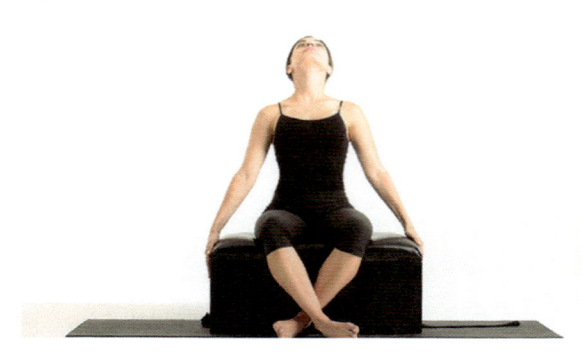

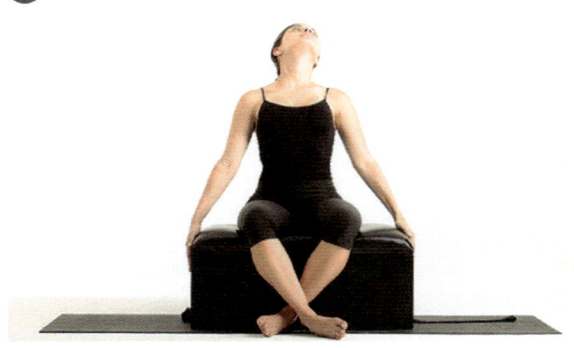

Ⓐ

Ⓑ

VARIATIONS: Photos B and C
- Turn face fractionally to one side and then the other
- Place bottom row of teeth above top row (undershot bite pattern)

CAUTION: IF YOU EXPERIENCE DIZZINESS DURING THIS STRETCH STOP IMMEDIATELY

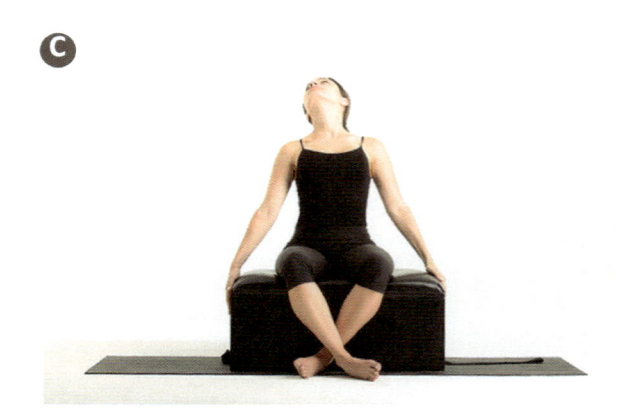

Ⓒ

Major muscles stretched
- Longus colli
- SCM
- Scalenus anterior

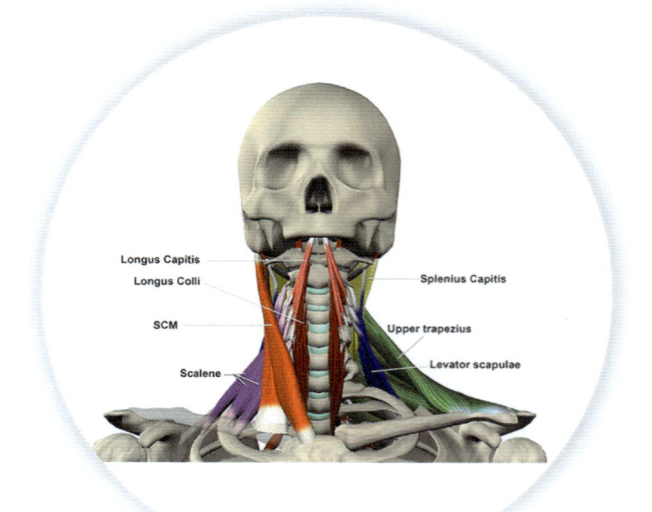

71 Jaw Extension

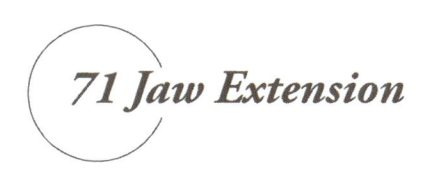

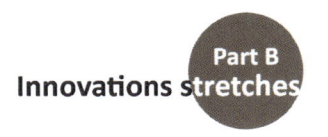

Part B
Innovations stretches

HOW TO STRETCH: Photos A and B
- Wash hands
- Sit in neutral position
- Open mouth and place two or three fingers on bottom front teeth
- Pull down on teeth to open mouth wider
- Clasp side of box for balance

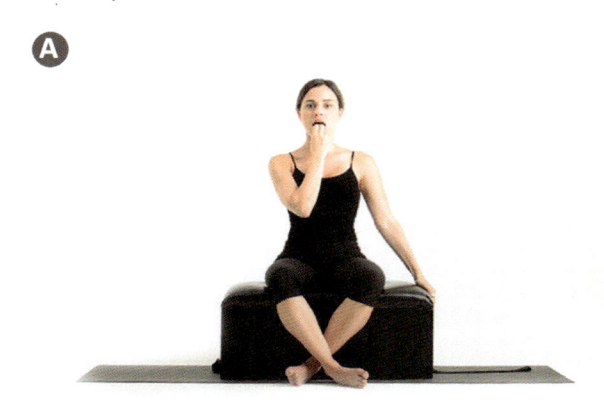

A

HOW TO CONTRACT: Photo B
- Press jaw up into fingers as if closing mouth

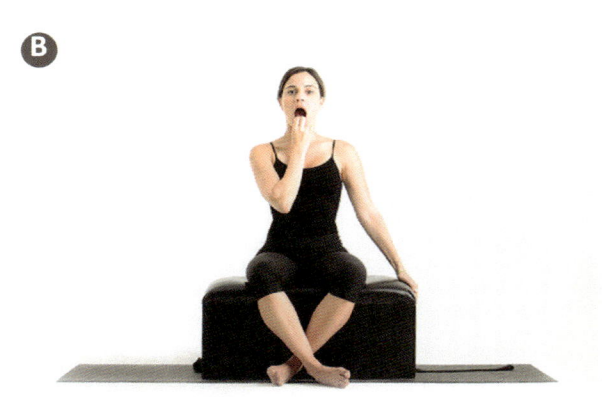

B

HOW TO RESTRETCH: Photos C and D
- Pull down further onto jaw and open mouth wider

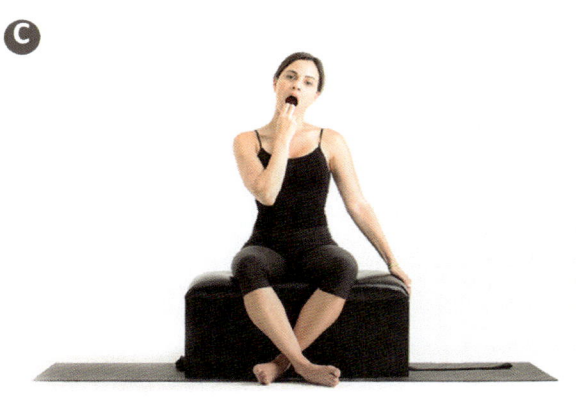

C

VARIATION: Photo D
- Pull down on jaw while tilting head left and right

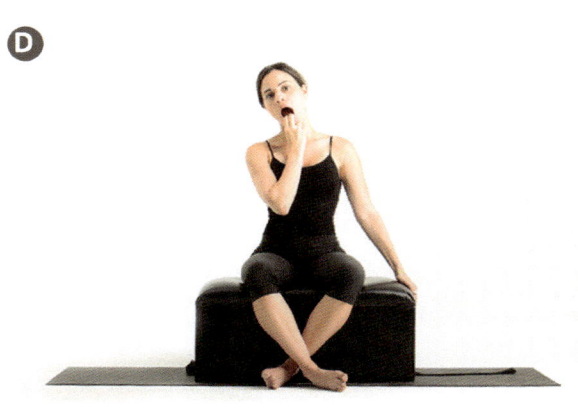

D

Major muscles stretched
Masseto
Temporalis

The Split
Chapter 9

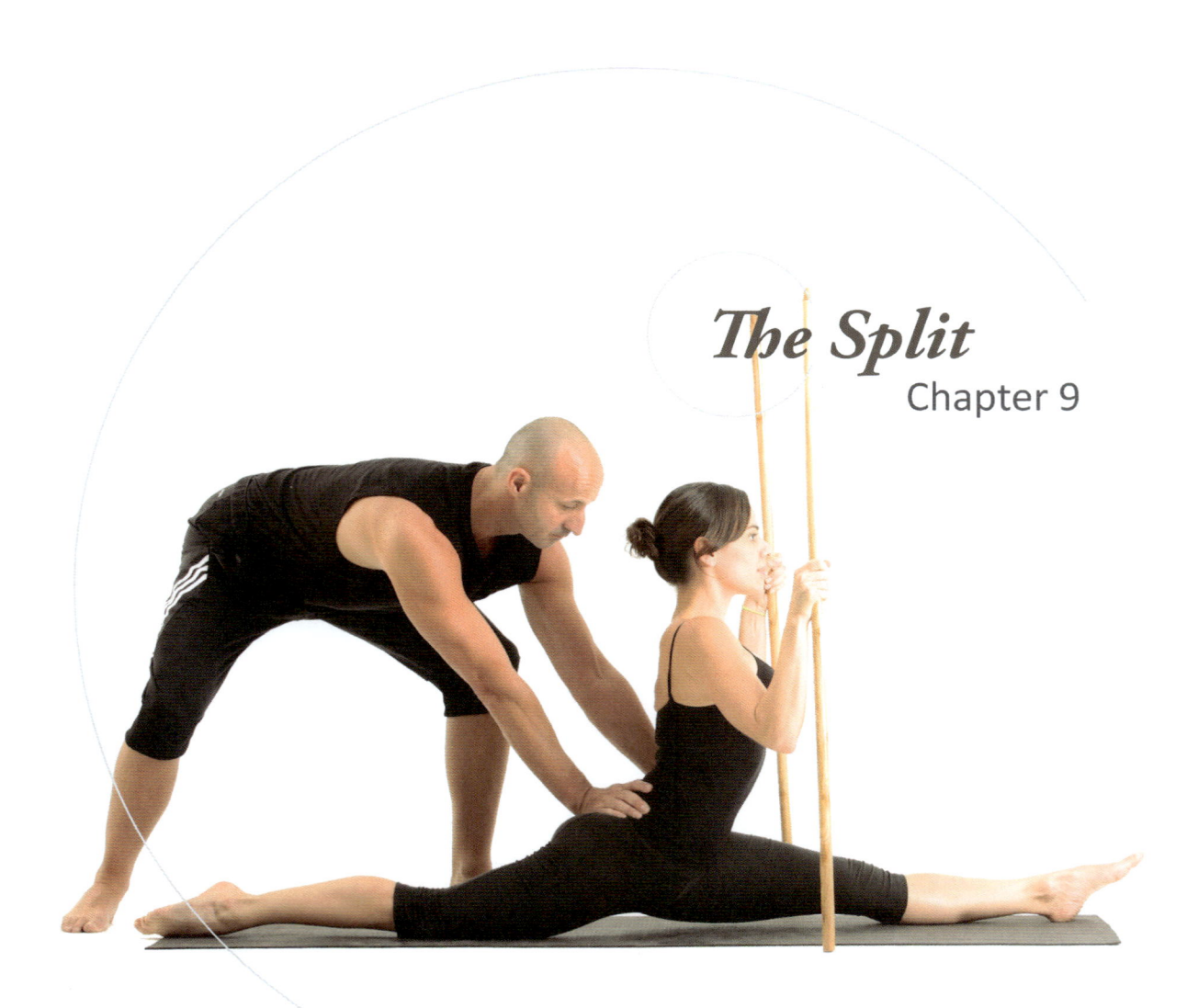

72 The Split

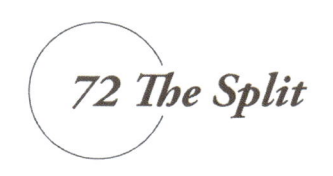

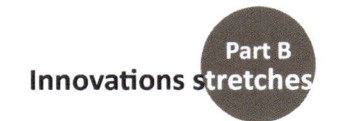

Part B — Innovations stretches

HOW TO STRETCH: Photo A
- Use two sticks for balance
- Press hands down into sticks to engage abdominals
- Slide legs apart to point of tension
- Lower hips as much as possible
- Partner to press down on sacrum to assist in holding neutral lumbar spine

HOW TO CONTRACT: Photo A
- Press knee of back leg and foot of front leg into floor

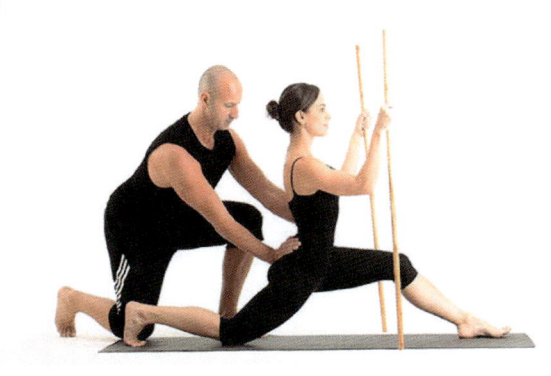

A

HOW TO RESTRETCH: Photo B
- Slowly slide legs apart and lower hips
- Maintain legs in parallel position
- Maintain neutral lumbar spine

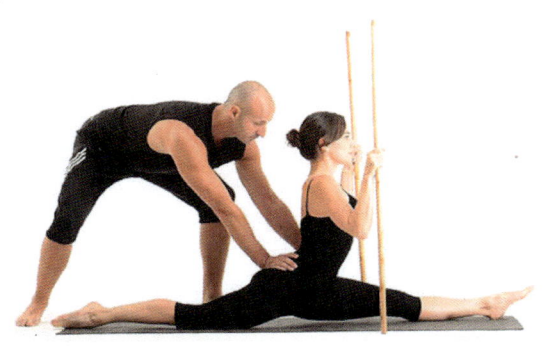

B

Major muscles stretched
- Hamstrings
- Iliopsoas
- Gluteus Maximus
- Adductor Magnus
- Rectus femoris
- Gastrocnemius

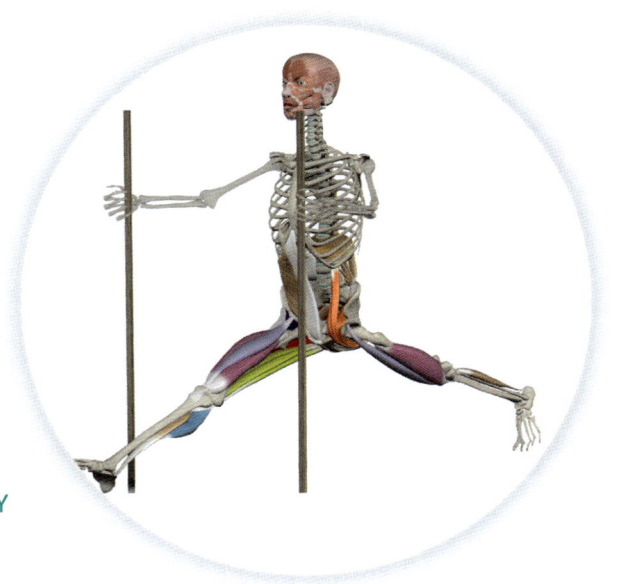

https://www.youtube.com/watch?v=wBC4Ozd2bqY

Some recommendations on how to use this book

Many of you will have enjoyed deepening your understanding of Pilates mat work while reading the deconstruction of each mat exercise contained in the book. You will have flicked from page to page, looking at the facilitating stretches and then the counterposes. In this section, we have attached an example of how you might simplify that process with the use of lesson charts called 'Innovations Application Charts'. You can refer to the sample below and then photocopy the blank tables that follow to create your own lesson plans. The tables you put together might be for your own reference, or they might form, for example, a ten-week course. You could decide that a complex exercise like the Wheel will be attempted on week ten of your course and place it accordingly. Some of the lesson time in the lead-up classes could be spent practising the facilitating stretches.

You can download free posters and charts from our Content Library at **www.innovationsinpilates.com**.

Innovations Application Charts

Pilates exercise		Facilitating stretches		Counterpose

Pilates exercise		Facilitating stretches		Counterpose

Pilates exercise		Facilitating stretches		Counterpose

Pilates exercise		Facilitating stretches		Counterpose

Concluding Comments

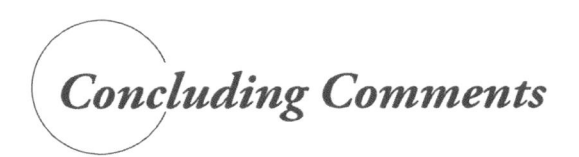

We truly hope you have enjoyed this book. It was (mostly!) a joy to write, though it took a little longer than expected with Kenyi and I busy teaching our material in over 25 countries. It's been a remarkable few years and we are delighted with the way the international Pilates community has embraced our work. Thank you to each and every person who has attended one of our workshops. There are dozens of postgraduate courses on offer, and dozens more ways to spend your weekends and income, so we are always appreciative when you choose to spend it with us.

The book started with the photo shoot in Caracas, Venezuela. Then Kenyi and I took time off between workshops and teaching at our Melbourne Studio to piece the content together over a two year period. We had writing time in Italy, Korea, London and then finally a week in Queensland, Australia, to finish it off. Once we got home to Melbourne, Australia, time was of the essence. With a baby due in four months, it was now or never!

Special thanks go to two wonderful people, Rael Isacowitz, owner of BASI Pilates, and Kristi Cooper, owner of Pilates Anytime. Both have been incredibly supportive and enthusiastic, embracing our work and helping share it with the Pilates community. We thank you sincerely.

The Pilates Method Alliance recognised the stretching aspect of Pilates as important and accredited all of our courses. For this we are grateful.

Gabriela Medina, of gabrielamedinaphoto.com, was terrific to work with. We shot thousands of pictures over two very long days. Thank you. We will come to your other studio in Paris for the next shoot.

Amit Alon, who has a unique story to tell, designed the fabulous graphic images for us. His material, called 'Muscle and Motion', is visually spectacular. Amit loves his work, and like us he also loves to educate, demystify and simplify so that people can understand what it is they are doing.

The beautiful Kenyi Diaz co-wrote and designed the entire book, as well as modelling all of the photographs with a little help from her friend Hilse Leon and myself. What a talented professional Kenyi is.

What's next? If you found benefit from our work, we hope you will come and study with us at one of our workshops or complete one of our certifications. It's when working together that the material found here really comes to life. Our reformer book is also due for a rewrite and our Anatomy for Pilates program will be released soon. So, lots to do, and lots to learn. We hope you will stay on the journey with us.

Take care, and stay loose.

Anthony and Kenyi

Bibliography

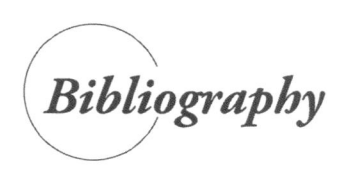

Ahearn, G. 2008. *General Anatomy: Principles and Applications*. McGraw Hill. Australia

Alter, MJ. 1996. *Science of Flexibility*. Human Kinetics. Australia.

Chaitow, L. 1988. *Soft Tissue Manipulation*. Healing Arts Press. Rochester, Vermont.

Coulter, HD. 2002. *Anatomy of Hatha Yoga*. Body and Breath. Honesdale, USA.

Frederick, A, and Frederick, C. 2006. *Stretch to Win*. Human Kinetics. Australia.

Grilley, P. 2004. *Anatomy for Yoga*. http://www.pranamaya.com

Jerome, J. 1987. *Fitness Stretching*. Breakaway Books. NY.

Juhan, D. 1987. *Job's Body*. Station Hill Press. NY.

Kapandji, LA. 1974. *The Physiology of the Joints*. Volumes 1–3. Churchill Livingstone. Edinburgh.

Kendall, HO. 1971. *Muscles, Testing and Function*. 2nd Edition. Williams and Wilkins. Baltimore.

Knott, M, & Voss, DE. 1968. *Proprioceptive Neuromuscular Facilitation*. Harper and Row. NY.

Kurtz, T. 1994. *Stretching Scientifically*. Stadion Publishing. USA.

Lederman, A. 2014. *Therapeutic Stretching*. Human Kinetics. Australia.

Long, R. 2005. *The Key Muscles of Hatha Yoga*. Bhandhayoga Publications. USA.

Long, R. 2008. *The Key Poses of Hatha Yoga*. Bhandhayoga Publications. USA.

McAtee, RE. 2007. *Facilitated Stretching*. Human Kinetics. Australia.

Myers, TW. 2009. *Anatomy Trains*. Churchill Livingstone. Sydney.

Neuman, DA. 2002. *Kinesiology of the Musculoskeletal System*. Mosby. USA.

Norris, C. 2004. *The Complete Guide to Stretching*. A & C Black Publishers. London.

Pilates, J. 1934. *Your Health*. Presentation Dynamics. Copywrited and reprinted 1988. USA.

Pilates, J. 1945. *Pilates' Return to Life through Contrology*. Presentation Dynamics. Copywrited and reprinted 1998. USA.

Richardson, JHH. 1999. *Therapeutic Exercise for Spinal Segmental Stabilization in Low Back Pain*. Churchill Livingstone. Sydney.

Sahrmann, SA. 2002. *Diagnosis and Treatment of Movement Impairment Syndromes*. Mosby. USA.

Tsatsouline, P. 2001. *Relax into Stretch*. Dragon Door Publications. USA.

Thompson, F. 1994. *Manual of Structural Kinesiology*. Mosby. Sydney.

Ylinen, J. 2008. *Stretching Therapy*. Churchill Livingstone. Sydney

Innovations in Pilates provides a range of products and classes for you to engage in our work

Books

Innovations in Pilates: Therapeutic Muscle Stretching on the Pilates Reformer
The counterpart to the book you are reading now, our reformer book teaches you how to stretch your entire body using the Pilates reformer. The Pilates reformer is a beautiful tool for stretching and this book is the basis for our Reformer Teacher Training certification, taught worldwide. To view and order, visit www.innovationsinpilates.com.

Innovations in Pilates certifications

Our Basi Pilates certifications are recognised by Pilates associations internationally, and are available worldwide. Follow us on Facebook, or check out our website at **www.innovationsinpilates.com.au**.

Pilates Retreats

We offer retreats that include daily Pilates and Innovations in Pilates classes, meditation and food coaching at our retreat venue in Bali. We also offer teacher training certifications at our Bali venue. Our certifications are available in both mat and reformer versions and include a host of other activities.

For information visit our website at **www.pilatesretreats.com.au**.

Pilates Anatomy

We teach anatomy in clay, with a unique emphasis on Pilates exercise. Check out our website or request a course tailored to your group's requirements. Follow us on Facebook at www.facebook.com/pilatesanatomy

Facebook and Websites

Please check out our links for all the latest information and fun photos.

www.innovationsinpilates.com
www.innovationsinpilates.com.au
www.pilatesretreats.com.au
www.anthonylett.com.au
www.fitzroypilates.com.au
www.facebook.com/pilatesanatomy
www.facebook.com/anthony.lett1
www.facebook.com/pages/Innovations-in-Pilates
www.facebook.com/FitzroyPilatesStudio?ref=hl
www.kenyidiaz.com
www.facebook.com/kenyi13?fref=ts

Innovations in Pilates on the Universal Reformer

The beautiful images on the following pages are from the second edition of our reformer book, available soon. We have included them to give you a sneak peek, but more interestingly, to give you an impression of how the mat work translates to the Pilates reformer.

Several of the images have been brought to life by some 3D video animations of their performance. Check out the YouTube links and enjoy! Check in with us too, because there are more on the way!

https://www.youtube.com/watch?v=wBC4Ozd2bqY

This is the reformer version of **the splits exercise page 152.**

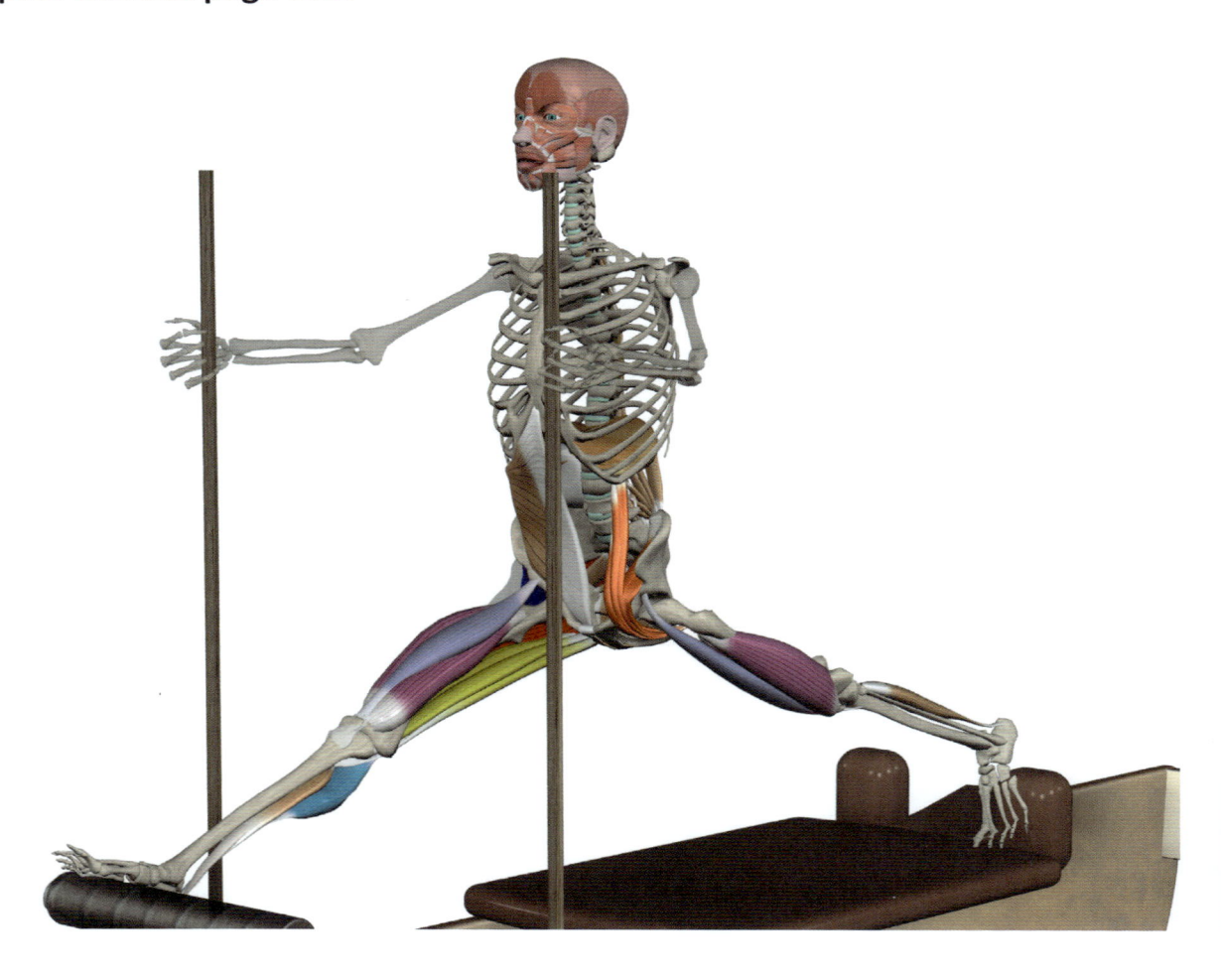

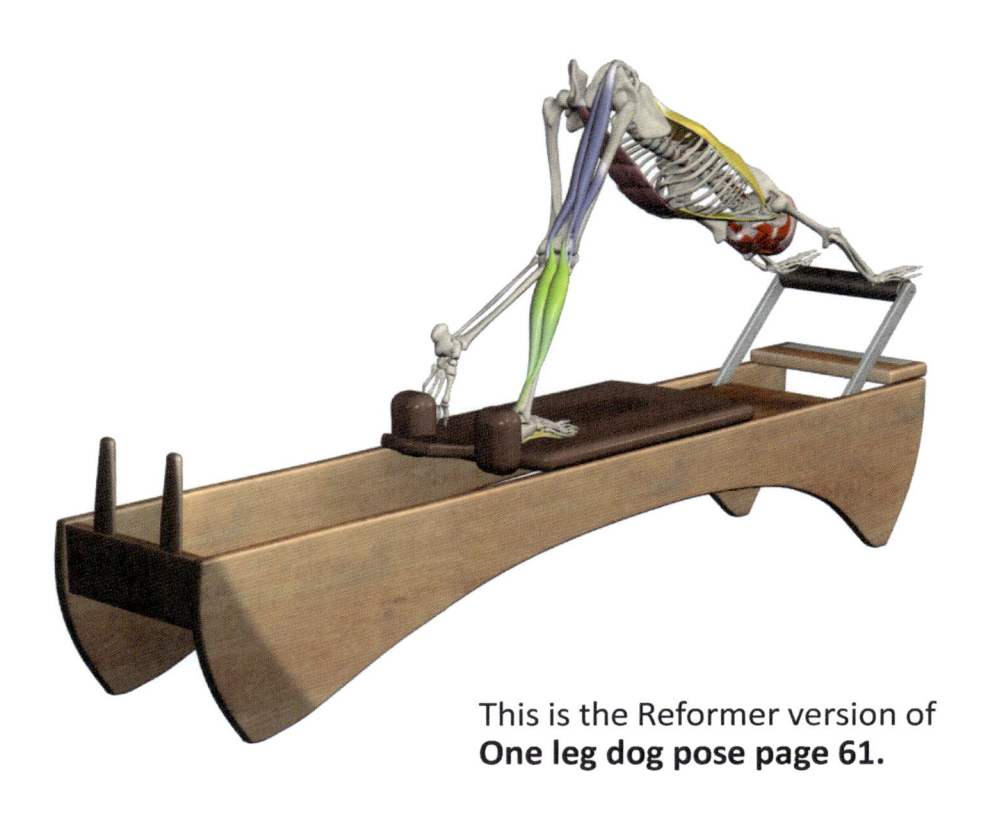

This is the Reformer version of **One leg dog pose page 61.**

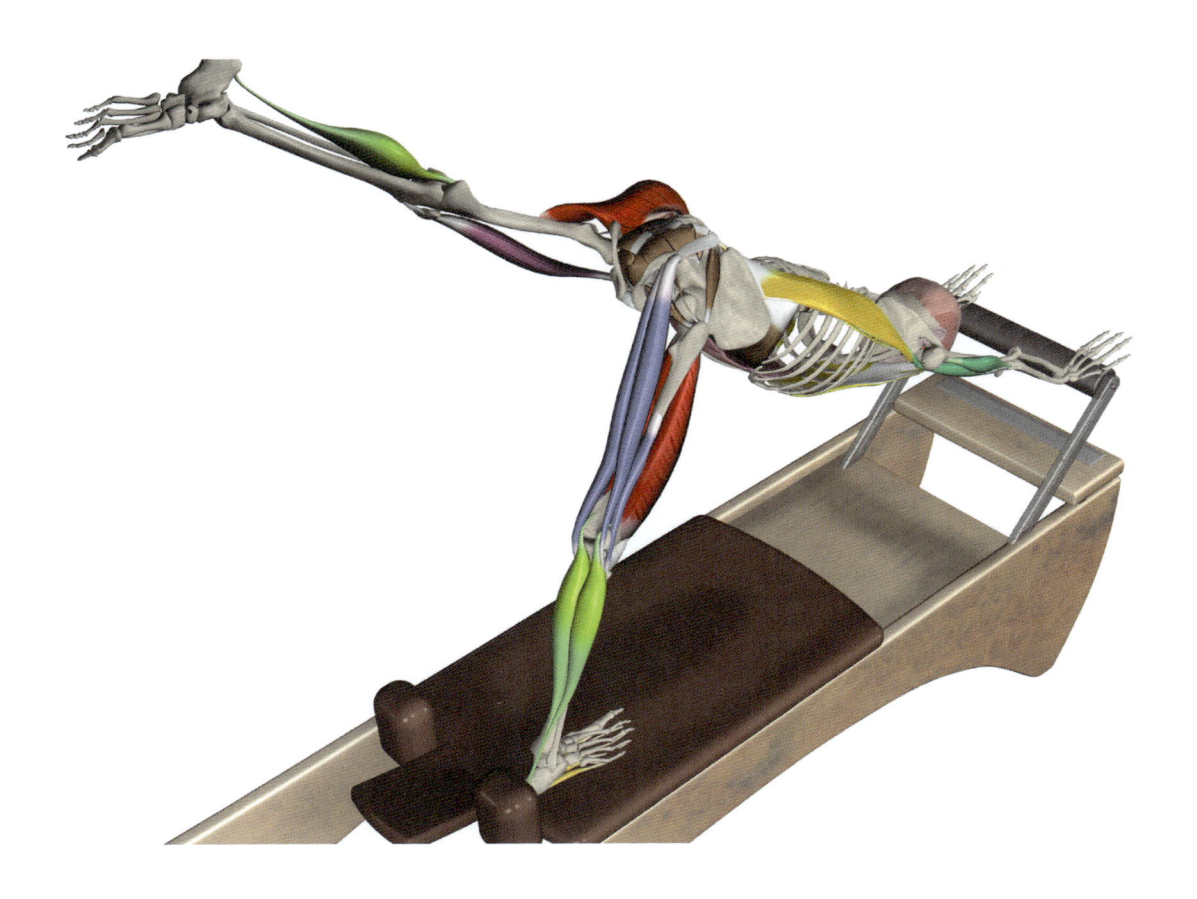

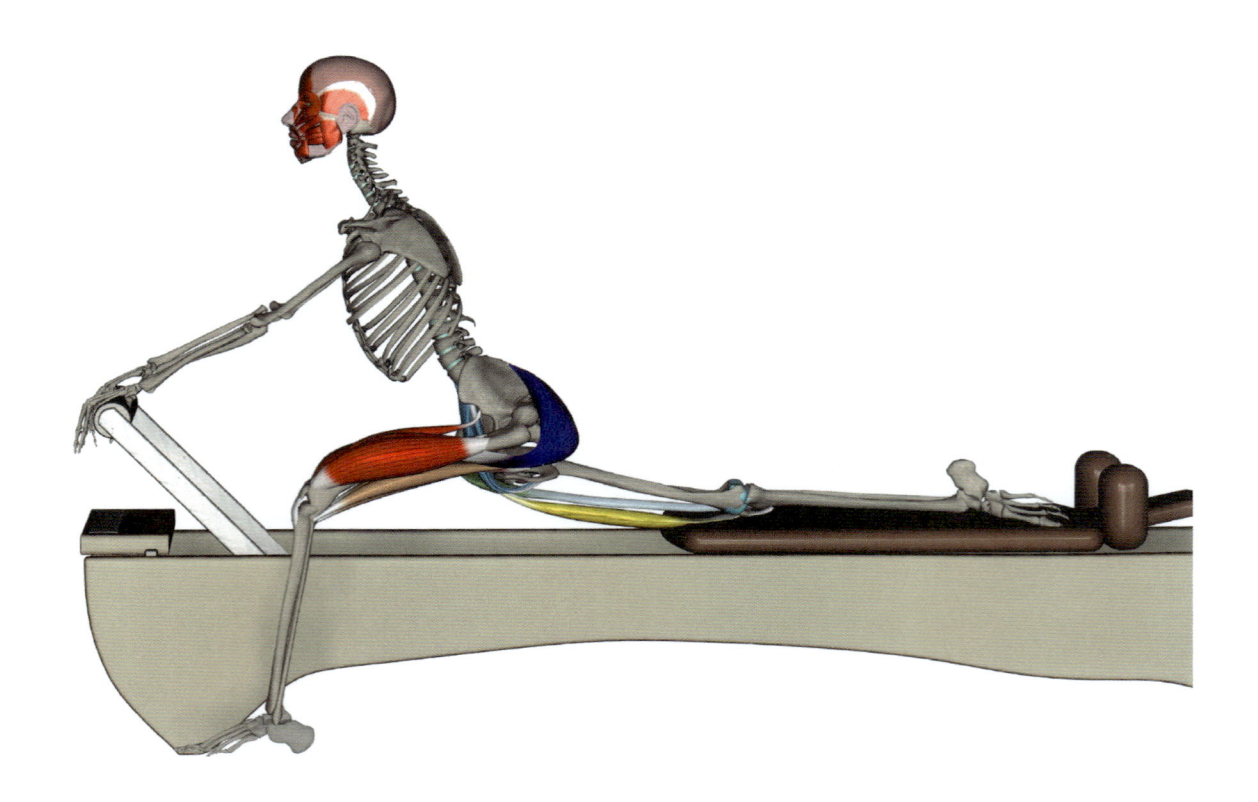

This is the Reformer version of **Kneeling Hip flexor stretch page 85.**

Check the dynamic video of this stretch

https://www.youtube.com/watch?v=-mIVVwA4vlc

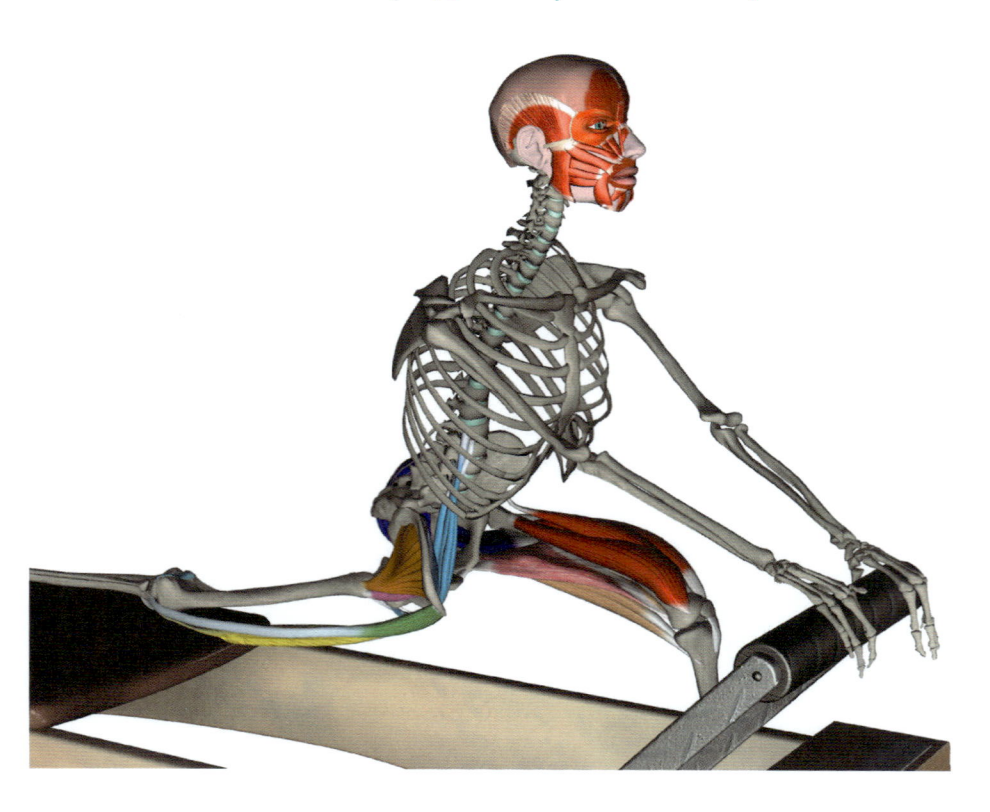

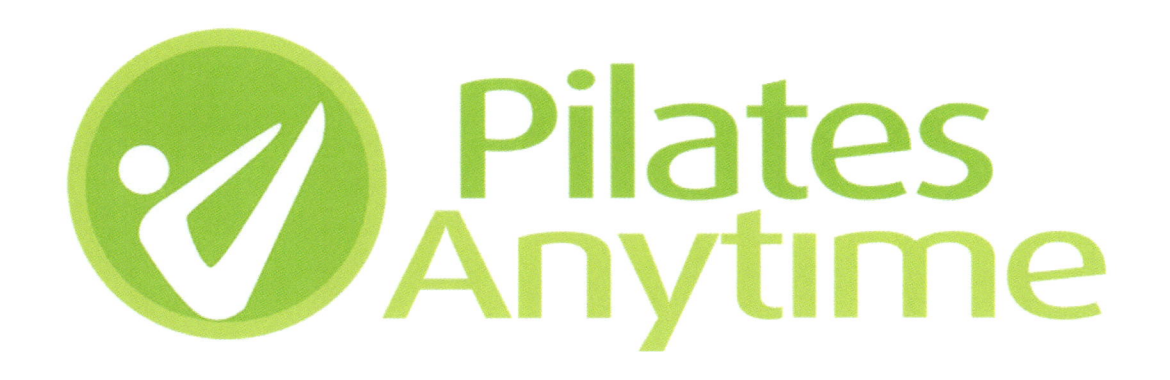

Innovations in Pilates has 12 classes on Pilates Anytime, the online resource with over 1,500 classes from the world's leading teachers. For a free one month subscription go to www.PilatesAnytime.com and enter the code 8752WPP.

We are proud to have worked closely with 'Muscle and Motion' on the graphic images in this book. Their resource is terrific for both Pilates instructions and anyone who works in physical or body-based therapies. To subscribe, visit their website and use the word 'Pilates' to receive a 20% discount. Highly recommended.

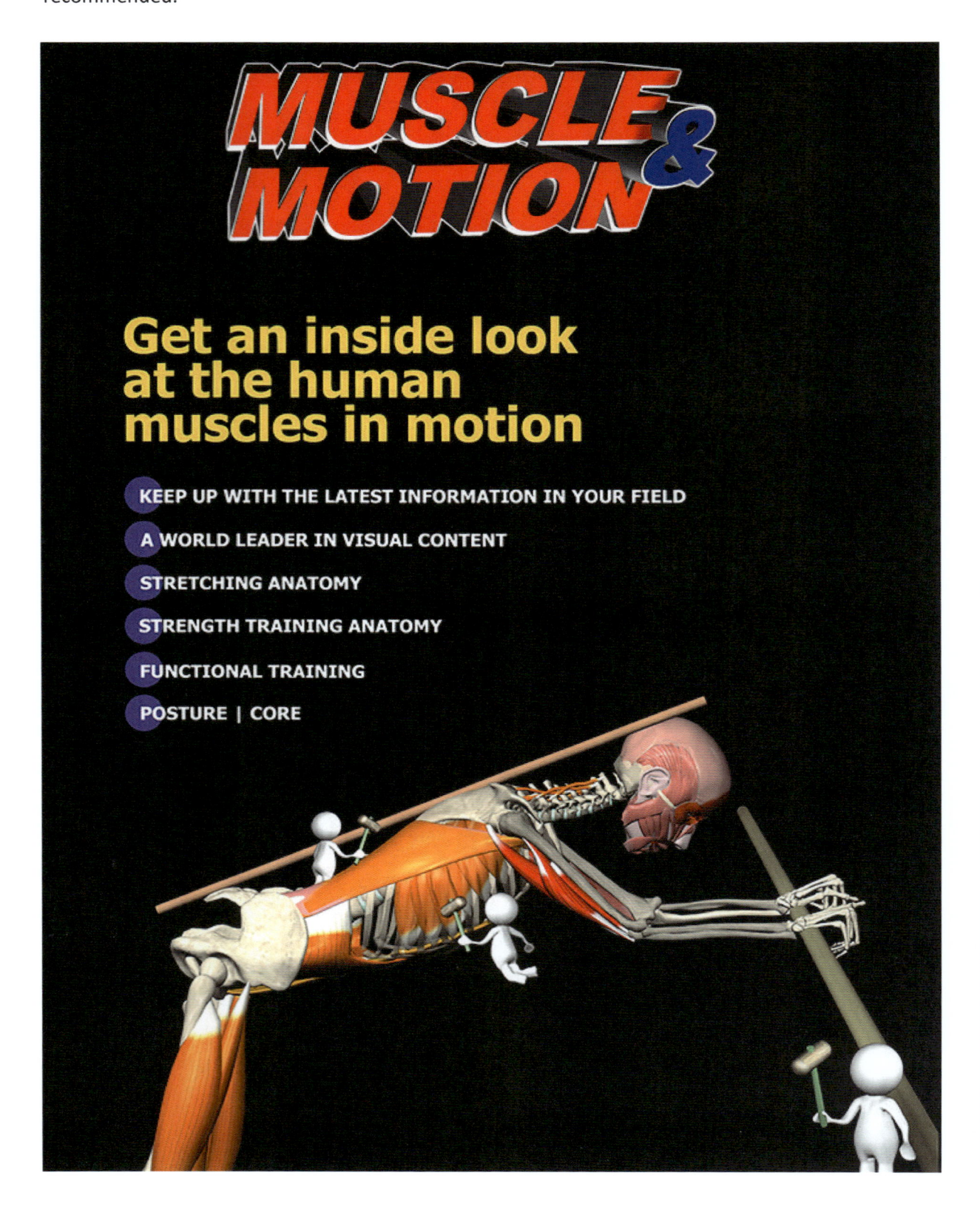

MUSCLE & MOTION

Get an inside look at the human muscles in motion

- KEEP UP WITH THE LATEST INFORMATION IN YOUR FIELD
- A WORLD LEADER IN VISUAL CONTENT
- STRETCHING ANATOMY
- STRENGTH TRAINING ANATOMY
- FUNCTIONAL TRAINING
- POSTURE | CORE

Printed in Great Britain
by Amazon